The Complete Family Guide to Living with High Blood Pressure

The Complete Family Guide to Living with High Blood Pressure

Michael K. Rees, M.D.

Drawings by Claudia Tarpley Rees

Prentice-Hall, Inc., Englewood Cliffs, New Jersey

10   9   8   7   6   5   4   3   2

Library of Congress Cataloging in Publication Data

Rees, Michael K
  The complete family guide to living with high blood pressure.

  Includes index.
  1. Hypertension.   2. Hypertension—Prevention.
I. Title. [DNLM: 1. Hypertension—Popular works.
WG340 R328c]
RC685.H8R38   616.1'32   80-18767
ISBN 0-13-160432-5

Contents

Acknowledgments

I would like to thank Susan and the boys for putting up with me during the writing of this book, Ms. Marylou Abbruzzese, R.D., who provided much helpful nutrition information, and the following physicians who were kind enough to review and comment upon various sections of the manuscript: Dr. Joseph Alpert, Department of Medicine, University of Massachusetts Medical School, Worcester, Mass.; Dr. Vicki Bernstein, Department of Medicine, Vancouver General Hospital, Vancouver, British Columbia; Dr. Robert Brown, Department of Medicine, Beth Israel Hospital, Boston, Mass.; Dr. Bryan Emmerson, Department of Medicine, Princess Alexandria Hospital, Queensland, Australia; Dr. Franklin Epstein, Department of Medicine, Beth Israel Hospital, Boston, Mass.; Dr. Emmanuel Friedman, Department of Obstetrics and Gynecology, Beth Israel Hospital, Boston, Mass.; and Dr. J. I. S. Robertson, MRC Blood Pressure Unit, Western Infirmary, Glasgow, Scotland. I have tried to the fullest extent possible to follow their good advice, but should there be any errors or omissions, the fault is entirely mine.

Author's Note

I believe that a doctor's first responsibility is to teach good health habits and that this is an even more important obligation than the ordering of tests and the dispensing of pills. A doctor must be committed to helping patients understand their health problems so that they can actively participate in their own care. To be truly effective, medicine must be a partnership. To be a partner means to be an equal, and to achieve this equality a patient must have the necessary information about major health issues.

True partnership between patient and doctor is especially important in the treatment of high blood pressure, an extremely common condition which may affect as many as one out of every six people living in our salt-eating Western society. Indeed, few societies anywhere in the world are spared this serious health problem which afflicts children and adults alike. Fortunately the measurement of blood pressure is painless and simple, the numbers which define it as high are well known, and high blood pressure is one of the easiest ailments to correct. The problem lies in the fact that although treatment is highly effective, high blood pressure can only be successfully managed by the patient because it requires a long term commitment to therapy. "Long term" in this case means every day, not just the days that happen to coincide with a visit to the doctor.

In my own medical practice it has been extremely frustrating to see how often my patients stop taking their blood pressure medication. Since they don't feel sick, why should they bother to swallow a pill? Over the years I have come to realize that the only way that I could convince patients to stick with their medication was to help them convince themselves that consistent therapy was in their best interest. Because I could not find the kind of reading material which I felt would allow patients to make an intelligent decision about the potential benefits of high blood pressure therapy, I decided to gather the information myself.

In the following pages, I have attempted to evaluate all that the experts have to say about high blood pressure and to present the facts clearly and fairly. After all, it's your body and you are entitled to know how you can best take care of it. I hope that after reading this book you will be as convinced as I am that if your blood pressure or the blood pressure of a member of your family is found to be elevated, a long-term commitment to therapy is a must.

Introduction

High blood pressure should always be treated. At one time doctors thought it was normal for our blood pressure to go up as we grow older. This is now known to be false. Extensive studies clearly show that our blood pressure should remain within normal range throughout life and that even the smallest rise in blood pressure above that level is a serious health hazard.

Until recently, doctors were not sure what numbers defined high blood pressure. Now they know—and you will learn exactly what these numbers are and how they were decided upon when you read Chapter 3. When you think about it, it's easy to understand how a small increase in blood pressure can be a major health hazard. Suppose your pressure rises slightly when you are 35 years of age. By the time you are 45, your heart, kidneys, and arteries have had to contend with an elevated pressure for 10 years. By age 55, they have been subjected to increased pressure for 20 years. It's not surprising that a heart that has to work against even a small increase in pressure for 10 or 20 years can get tired or that arteries to the brain which are constantly forced to carry blood at even a slightly increased pressure can develop wear and tear of their walls, making them susceptible to rupture. After consistent exposure to even a mild elevation in pressure, it's no wonder that the arteries to the kidneys can stiffen and become less capable of filtering and purifying the blood or that there is an increased associated tendency to push cholesterol and fat into the walls of the arteries, leading to the buildup of deposits which can in turn create blockage of the circulation. Clearly, control of high blood pressure, no matter how small the elevation, is one of the most important health measures we can take.

Doctors now know that the number of deaths from heart disease and stroke can be approximately cut in half when blood pressure is adequately treated. These are mortality statistics. It takes longer to develop the statistics which tell just how much illness—as opposed to death—is prevented when high blood pressure is controlled, but data is coming in. It is already clear that approximately one half of all cases of stroke and one third of all cases of heart disease can be eliminated through effective blood pressure management. No doubt, within a few years, the data will similarly document that a large percentage of all cases of kidney failure and circulatory disease can be entirely avoided simply by treating high blood pressure. Since most individuals have "mild" high blood pressure, you can be sure that the data will also show that the most impressive results are obtained by correcting small elevations of blood pressure, the kind of numbers which until a few years ago, many doctors neglected to treat.

If you don't know what your blood pressure numbers are, find out. It takes less than a minute to measure blood pressure, and the technique involved is painless and simple. A doctor is not required. You can easily learn to measure your own blood pressure and the blood pressure of other members of your family. If you learn that your blood pressure numbers are out of range, insist on treatment. Your doctor will begin therapy by recommending salt restriction and, if you are overweight, weight reduction. It is estimated that about one half of all cases of high blood pressure can be cured by these two measures alone, but if they do not bring your pressure completely within normal range, a medication will be advised. Of those who need medication, more than half can be successfully treated by a single medicine taken once daily.

Once a diagnosis has been made and treatment decided upon, the rest is up to you. Only you can eliminate excess salt from your diet, keep your weight at normal range and be faithful to your medication, should medication be necessary. But in order to effectively participate in the treatment of a high blood pressure condition in this and other ways there are a number of things you need to know. It is the purpose of this book to give you that information.

You will learn, for example, that the accurate measurement of blood pressure requires the right equipment, the right surroundings, and proper technique. You certainly don't want to be treated for high blood pressure if your pressure is normal; nor do you want to be told that your blood pressure is normal if it is in fact elevated. Before further steps are taken, you must insist that the procedures outlined in Chapter 2 are followed.

You will learn that eliminating excess salt from your diet is not as simple as it sounds. The highest amount of salt is often contained in foods that don't taste at all salty. Specific instructions about proper diet are given in chapters 8 and 16.

You will learn how blood pressure medication can lead to a potassium deficiency which the proverbial daily banana alone will not control. How to maintain a healthy potassium level is discussed in Chapter 8.

You will learn in Chapter 7 to identify the three different groups of medicines used to treat high blood pressure and the peculiarities as well as the common side effects of all the blood pressure medicines employed throughout the world.

You will learn about the areas of special concern for women: whether to use either the contraceptive pill or the female hormone, estrogen, if you have high blood pressure; how to protect not only your own health but that of your developing baby if you are pregnant; what to do about breast feeding. These issues are dealt with in chapters 10 through 12.

You will learn what special steps a parent with high blood pressure must take to protect a child. As important as it is to detect and treat high blood pressure in adults, it is even more vital that this be accomplished in children. The important diagnostic and preventive health measures with which you should be familiar are fully explained in Chapter 13.

You will learn that certain forms of exercise activity may bring a small elevation of blood pressure down to normal and eliminate the need for medication. Others, however, are potentially dangerous. Which forms of exercise you should choose are discussed in Chapter 14 along with forms of blood pressure medicine to be used with extreme caution if you are physically very active.

You will learn how to monitor your own blood pressure or that of a family member by purchasing your own blood pressure kit. Chapter 15 will show you how to choose such equipment and provide you with full instructions for its use.

These are only a few of the topics covered in this complete family guide to the prevention and treatment of high blood pressure. As you read through the following pages remember that everyone who has high blood pressure should have the opportunity to lead a full and productive life, free not only from the potentially harmful effects of the disease itself but from the possibly troublesome side effects of the medicines employed in its treatment. You and your family are entitled to the very best of medical care. This book is dedicated to giving you the necessary information to make that right a reality.

The Complete Family Guide to Living with High Blood Pressure

1

WHAT IS BLOOD PRESSURE?

When you stand on your head, how does blood get to your feet? Answer: blood pressure. When you stand on your feet, why isn't your brain deprived of its blood supply? Same answer. Water can't flow uphill and neither can blood. It takes pressure to force water upward—water pressure—and a water pump is required to create this pressure. Similarly, it takes pressure to force blood to all the parts of your body—blood pressure—and this pressure is created by a blood pump, your heart.

It sediment builds up in a water pipe, the inside of the pipe becomes narrowed. When this happens, the water pump must work harder to force water through the pipe. The pump must create greater pressure to keep the liquid flowing. As the opening within the pipe becomes smaller and smaller, the pump has to generate more and more pressure to keep the liquid moving. Eventually, if something isn't done to unclog the pipe, one of two things may happen. The pump may have to force water through the pipe under such a high pressure that the pipe must burst and cause a flood. Or the pump may just stop working.

Your heart is a pump. Its job is to pump blood through the intricate network of blood vessels which make up your circulation. The heart is a hollow muscle, something like a balloon. It expands as it fills up with blood, and then it contracts and forces the blood out through blood vessels, which are called *arteries*. How hard must the heart work? That depends upon the condition of the arteries. If the arteries are in good shape, there is less work for the heart to do. Your heart is not lazy, but it has to last a lifetime. It has to make sure that every part of your body has an adequate blood supply, whether you are standing on your feet or standing on your head.

The lower the blood pressure, the better, just so long as blood gets to where it has to go. The lower the pressure, the less work for the heart.

Blood pressure reflects the force with which your heart

pushes blood through the arteries. Does *all* the pressure come from the pumping action of your heart? The answer is no. The heart creates pressure when it pumps, but it doesn't pump all the time. The heart rests while it fills up with blood, and during this resting time it does not create any pressure.

What happens to your circulation while your heart is filling with blood? Is there still pressure in the blood vessels? It is important for you to know the answers to these two questions so that you can understand how your doctor measures your blood pressure. A clue to these answers lies in the fact that blood pressure measurements consist of two numbers.

Suppose you are told that your blood pressure is 140 over 80? What does this mean? The top number, 140, is easy to understand. That is the pressure in the pipe when the heart is pushing on the blood to force it through the circulation. In Chapter 2 you will see exactly how this is measured. What about the lower number, 80? Since the heart does not create pressure while resting, shouldn't the lower number be zero between beats? Visualizing the following experiment should clarify what happens in the blood vessels while the heart is resting:

Imagine that you have a small glass tube. Now fill it with water so that no empty space is left. Then tightly seal both ends of the tube. Turn the tube upside down. What happens? Nothing. Why? Because no matter how you position it, the tube remains completely full of liquid. Liquid continues to touch all of its walls.

Now open up one end of the tube, let out half of the water, and reseal the tube. Turn the tube upside down. What happens? The water runs down the tube, filling the bottom half and leaving the top half empty. Only the walls of the bottom half of the tube are in contact with the liquid.

Now lay the tube on a table. What does the water do? It spreads evenly throughout the tube so that there is a layer of water from one end to the other, but now there is no liquid touching the upper wall.

Now imagine that your arteries are glass tubes and that they are entirely filled with blood. Whether you stand up, sit down, lie down, or bend over, the glass arteries remain filled up with blood. There is no problem of empty spaces. But suppose you decide to be a good citizen and donate a pint of blood to the blood bank. What happens then? You have let some of the liquid out of the tubes, leaving them only partially filled. If you lie down, blood is still present from one end to the other. But suppose you stand up. The tops of the glass tubes are now empty. The top of your body is suddenly without blood!

How can this problem be solved? How must your blood

vessels be engineered so that they remain constantly filled with blood? How can you be sure that no matter what your position, all parts of your body maintain a blood supply? Answer: *Make the walls elastic.*

Let's look at the advantage of elastic blood vessels. If the walls of a tube are flexible, then it is possible always to have liquid entirely filling the tube no matter how little liquid is present. The inside of the tube is adaptable. When there is a lot of liquid, the tube is wide. When there is less liquid, the tube is narrow. The advantage of this arrangement is that no matter how you position the tube, there are no empty spaces.

This is how your blood vessels work. If you drink a lot of liquid and increase the volume of your blood, the blood vessels can expand. If you don't drink sufficient liquid or if you donate blood and decrease its volume, the blood vessels can contract. When you change position, the walls of your blood vessels press in on the blood to keep it in place and in this way prevent any part of the blood vessels from becoming empty. The elastic tension in the walls of the arteries causes them to press on the blood. They create pressure on the blood. Even when your heart is not pumping, your blood is under the pressure created by the elastic tension in the walls of your blood vessels. *This pressure of the walls of the arteries pushing on the blood is the other component of blood pressure.* This is what the bottom number of the blood pressure measurement refers to.

Now you know what the two numbers that measure blood pressure represent. The top number gives the pressure in your circulation when the heart is beating with maximum effort to force the blood through the blood vessels. The bottom number is the pressure in the circulation when the heart is filling between beats. Now you know why blood doesn't drain from your feet when you stand on your head or drain from your head when you stand on your feet.

Your blood pressure is influenced not only by the condition of the insides of the pipes—the extent to which the arteries are or are not clogged—but also by the elasticity of the walls of the arteries. Just as it is less work for your heart to push blood through arteries that are unclogged and nicely open, it is also less work to push blood through soft, flexible arteries than through arteries that have lost some of their elasticity. Normally the walls of the arteries are elastic: They yield when blood is pushed through them by the pumping action of the heart. If the vessels become stiff and no longer widen easily when the heart beats, more work is created for the heart. This is why you want to keep your arteries as soft and as flexible as possible. It is one of the reasons for watching your diet. Reducing your fat and cholesterol consumption will lessen the danger of deposits inside the arterial walls which make the arteries stiff.

The purpose of blood pressure is to ensure that all parts of your body receive an adequate supply of blood at all times, whatever your posture or body motion. Blood pressure is measured by two numbers. The top number represents the pressure in the circulation when the heart is pushing on the blood to force it to all parts of the body. The bottom number represents the pressure in the arteries when the heart is filling with blood between beats.

THE BLOOD PRESSURE CONTROL SYSTEM

The blood pressure control system will be discussed in more detail in Chapter 6, but it will be helpful if you have a brief understanding now of how the system operates.

Three machines in the body—the *heart*, the *kidneys*, and the *arteries*—work together to keep your blood pressure normal. They can raise or lower your pressure in the following ways:

1. The *heart* may pump more forcefully or less forcefully. If the heart pumps with greater force, the blood pressure goes up, and if the heart pumps with less force, the blood pressure goes down.

2. The *kidneys* can retain or lose salt and water. If the kidneys retain salt and water, this excess fluid collects in the tissues all through the body and stretches them. When blood is pumped by the heart, it is forced first into the arteries, then out into the tissues to deliver oxygen and food throughout the body. The blood then returns to the heart through an entirely different set of pipes called *veins*. You know that if the arteries become stiff, the heart must work harder. The tissues can also become stiff. If this occurs, it becomes more difficult for the blood to leave the arteries, flow into the tissues, and then return to the veins. What can make the tissues stiff? Stretching due to the excess salt and water deposited there by the kidneys. At times, so much stretching may occur that it takes the form of visible swelling—puffy ankles, puffy eyes, or puffy hands. Usually, the amount of excess fluid is not this great and you will not be able to detect its presence on your own. However, your heart can tell when such extra fluid accumulates because it will have to work harder. The stiff tissues create a resistance to the flow of the blood out of the arteries, and blood pressure goes up.

If the kidneys get rid of the salt and water, the blood pressure will go down. When the tissues are not stretched by salt and water, they can receive the blood from the arteries with less resistance. Since it is now easier for the heart to pump blood into the tissues, the blood pressure goes down.

3. The *arteries* can become wider or narrower. The arteries have walls which contain muscles and elastic tissue. We have seen how the walls of the arteries actually push in on the blood within them, and how they can do this with a lot of pressure or with a little pressure. It is important that the arteries have this elastic quality, because it is by being elastic that they are able to stay full at all times. Remember the example of the glass tube. The walls of the arteries are elastic because they actually have tissue in them that has elastic properties and also because the walls of the arteries contain muscles which can expand and contract to make the openings of the arteries either larger or smaller. When the inside of the arteries is made smaller, the heart has to push harder on the blood to force it through the narrowed arteries and blood pressure goes up. There is also more pressure in the arteries themselves because the walls of the arteries push on the blood with more pressure.

If the muscles in the arteries relax and are less stiff, there is less pressure on the blood within the arteries. Also, because the arteries are more relaxed and easier to distend, it is easier for the heart to pump blood through them, and as a result the blood pressure goes down.

THE COMMUNICATION NETWORK OF THE BLOOD PRESSURE CONTROL SYSTEM

The heart, the kidneys, and the arteries all work together to try to keep your blood pressure normal at all times. If one part of the system makes the blood pressure go too high, the other parts of the system will compensate to bring the pressure back to normal. If one part of the system makes the blood pressure fall too low, the other parts of the system will compensate to bring the system back up to normal. Your body is equipped with a communication system to ensure that the three machines of the blood pressure system work together smoothly and effectively. Your nervous system is an important part of this blood pressure communication network.

Before we go on to discuss blood pressure control in more detail, you need to know how blood pressure is measured. Also you need to know how you can be certain that your blood pressure is always measured accurately. These topics will be discussed in the next two chapters.

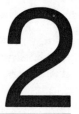

HOW BLOOD PRESSURE IS MEASURED

If you stand by a stream and shut your eyes, how can you tell if the water in the stream is moving without touching the water? If you can't see the water and if you can't touch the water, what *can* you do? You can *hear* the water. The same principal applies in blood pressure measurement.

Unless the walls of a stream are extremely smooth, you will be able to distinguish rippling sounds as the water flows over the rocks and branches that interrupt its flow. If the stream is moving very slowly, the sounds will be very soft. You will have to listen very carefully to hear them; you may have to bend over and place your ear close to the edge of the stream. If the stream is flowing very rapidly, the sound of the flowing water may be quite loud and easy to hear. Either way, with your eyes closed and without touching the water, you will be able to tell that the water is moving. Only two things are required: there must be something in the stream which interferes with the flow of the water so that it makes a rippling noise, and there must be some way for you to hear that rippling sound. If the sound is very soft, it may be necessary for you to use some sort of special listening device, one that amplifies sound. Your doctor's stethoscope is such an amplifier; it makes soft sounds louder and easier to hear.

What do flowing streams have to do with determining blood pressure? If you look at the way your doctor measures your blood pressure, this will become clear. The first thing your doctor does is to wrap a device around your arm called a blood pressure cuff. It is simply a piece of cloth with a rubber bag inside it. When the cloth is securely in place, your doctor pumps air into the rubber bag. The cloth cover and the rubber bag are especially constructed so that when the rubber bag inside the cuff expands with air, your muscles and fatty tissues are squeezed by the air pressure from the pump.

What does this squeezing process accomplish? The doctor's aim is to apply enough pressure to the artery bringing blood to the arm so that the arterial walls touch each other and the blood flow is stopped. Now the measurement-taking can begin. It works this way: A little pressure is let out of the rubber bag, just enough to allow a slight opening in the artery. We now have the situation of a stream with rocks protruding into the water, the rocks in this case being the sides of the artery. Blood can now flow again, but it makes a noise as it passes over the indented sides of the tube.

The blood pressure cuff is connected to a gauge which shows exactly how much pressure is being applied to your arm. As the pressure in the cuff is slowly released, the doctor stands by the bank of the stream and waits for the first noise of flowing blood, which will come as soft tapping sounds. Since the sound of the stream is very soft, the doctor holds a stethoscope as close to the side of the stream as possible. It is placed just below the junction of the upper arm and the forearm and slightly left of center, directly above the artery known as the *brachial artery*. The stethoscope amplifies the tapping sounds. When the very first sound is heard, the doctor knows that the pressure in the cuff is just below the pressure necessary to completely stop the flow of blood. While listening for these sounds, the doctor carefully watches the pressures gauge of the blood pressure cuff. *The number that appears on the pressure gauge just as the first sound is heard is the top number of the blood pressure.*

The top number of the blood pressure, then, is the maximum pressure that is required to push the blood and move it through the arteries. This number is measured by applying enough pressure on the artery to completely stop the flow of blood and then standing by the bank of the stream and listening for the first tapping noise as the pressure is carefully lowered.

How is the bottom number of your blood pressure reading determined? As the pressure of the cuff upon the artery is very carefully lowered, the "rocks and branches" of the arterial wall become smaller and smaller. Since there is less interference with the flow of the stream, the sounds your doctor will hear become softer and softer. Finally, there will be no sound at all. Your doctor keeps carefully watching the gauge as the pressure is being lowered. *The number that appears on the gauge just as the sounds disappear is the lower number of your blood pressure.* This is the pressure which the elastic walls of the arteries exert on the blood when the heart is filling up between beats. It is the pressure in the circulation between heartbeats.

What does it mean when you are told that your pressure is, for example, 120 over 80? It means that the first sound was heard at a pressure reading of 120 and that the last sound was heard at a pressure reading of 80. Both numbers are equally important. The top number is the maximum force that the heart must apply to make sure blood gets to every place it must go. The bottom number is the initial pressure which the heart must work against as it sends blood through the system. It is in the heart's best interest to have as little starting resistance to pump against as possible. The less pressure the heart must exert to get the blood distributed throughout the circulation, the better.

What constitutes normal, high, and low blood pressure will be discussed later. For the moment, the important thing to know is that both numbers in a blood pressure reading are equally important and that both must be measured accurately.

Since it is necessary to pick up extremely soft sounds to determine both the top and bottom numbers of your blood pressure, mistakes can easily be made. As we have seen, in measuring the top number it is necessary to determine when the sound *first* appears. The examiner slowly releases the pressure in the cuff around your arm while listening with the stethoscope and watching the blood pressure gauge. If the person measuring your pressure isn't extremely careful, the top number may be thought to be *lower* than it actually is. It is like riding in a car and looking for the number of a house. The house you want is 136 Elm Street. Your teenager is driving the car while you look for the correct number. Not every house is clearly marked. You see 168, 164, 156, 150, 146. You suggest slowing down because you are almost there. But you know how teenagers are! 142, 140, 128 ... whoops! ... you've gone too far!

When you are looking for a house, mistakes such as this don't really much matter. You can always turn around and try again. But when someone is looking for your blood pressure number, there is no advance way of knowing what the correct number is. Is it 136 or is it 128? If the person measuring your blood pressure goes past 136 without hearing it and first hears, say, 128, what is the result? You are told that the top number of your blood pressure is *lower* than it actually is.

To measure the bottom number of your blood pressure, it is necessary to hear the *last* sound. The noises get softer and softer as the pressure in the blood pressure cuff is released. The examiner keeps watching the pressure gauge while *slowly* releasing the pressure to make sure when that *last* sound is actually heard. You can imagine how easy it is to stop too soon, to think that you have heard the last ripple when a faint gurgle or two still remain. If this happens, you will be told that the bottom number of your blood pressure is *higher* than it really is.

To measure blood pressure accurately, good hearing and good equipment are essential. The blood pressure cuff valve must be able to be adjusted so that the pressure can be released slowly and evenly. The stethoscope must be able to adequately amplify soft sounds. The person measuring the pressure must be very careful and very patient.

There is another way that the top number can be measured, and that is the touch or *palpation* method. This is not as accurate as the method explained above but it is easier and it gives a reasonable estimate of the top number. We know that the blood vessels are elastic. When blood is pushed through the elastic artery and causes a pulse beat, the artery expands like a balloon. You can usually feel this expansion without equipment of any kind. You need only place the tips of your first and second fingers lightly on the inside of your wrist just below the base of your thumb. If the artery that supplies blood to this part of your wrist is squeezed closed, no blood can get to your wrist; therefore, the pulse cannot be felt.

As we have seen, the top number of your blood pressure measurement reflects the pressure with which the heart is pumping blood out into the circulation. Your doctor can get a good idea of this number through the palpation method by raising the pressure in the blood pressure cuff while keeping the fingers on the spot of your wrist where your pulse is felt. The pressure in the cuff is continually raised until the pulse disappears, and then the pressure is carefully lowered while watching the numbers on the pressure gauge. As soon as the doctor can first feel your pulse again, the pressure on the gauge is recorded. This will be a close approximation of the top number. It will be slightly lower than the true number, which is obtained with the aid of a stethoscope. There is a simple reason for this. The palpation method relies on touch rather than hearing and our fingers are not as sensitive as our ears.

In Chapter 15, complete instructions are provided in case you wish to learn how to measure your own blood pressure. There are a number of blood pressure measuring devices on the market, and the benefits and disadvantages of each type are discussed.

WHAT ABOUT THE NEW ELECTRONIC DEVICES THAT MEASURE BLOOD PRESSURE?

Electronic blood pressure machines measure blood pressure the same way that your doctor does, but instead of a stethoscope they substitute a speaker, a light, or a printing device. In the first case an electronic sound amplifier is connected to a speaker which is built into the blood pressure cuff and located so that it will lie approximately over the artery in the upper arm. The pressure in the blood pressure cuff is raised and then slowly lowered. As the first sound is heard and electronically amplified (top number), a beeping noise will begin. This beeping will stop when the sound disappears (bottom number). The sound amplifier can also be connected to a light in such a way that the light goes on when the sound is present and goes off when the sound stops. Again, the pressure in the blood pressure cuff is raised and then slowly lowered. When the first sound appears, a light will go on (top number), and the light will flash each time the tapping sound occurs. The light will permanently disappear when the sound disappears (bottom number). If the light is on a pressure dial, you can simply watch the dial and note the number on the dial when the light comes on and the number on the dial when the light permanently goes off. It is a way of "hearing" with your eyes.

The electronic blood pressure machine utilizing a printout is the most sophisticated of the three. These machines note the two blood pressure numbers on a piece of paper. They are too expensive for home use but may sometimes be found in drugstores, shopping malls, and other public places.

It is important to remember that none of these electronic machines is necessarily accurate and that you should *not* rely only on the readings from any one of them. The kinds of errors they can make and why will be discussed in the next chapter.

SYSTOLIC AND DIASTOLIC

Before we go on to discuss ways to be sure that your blood pressure is being accurately measured, there are two words with which you should familiarize yourself: *systolic* and *diastolic*.

Heart action has two phases, contraction and filling. You know that the top number of your blood pressure is the force with which the heart pushes on the blood to force it through the circulation. It is the pressure the heart pump exerts at the peak of its *contraction*. This *contraction phase* of heart action is called the *systolic phase*. The blood pressure at the peak of the contraction is called the *systolic blood pressure*. If your blood pressure is 120 over 80, then 120 is your systolic blood pressure.

After contracting, the heart rests and fills. This second phase of heart action is called the *diastolic phase*. We have seen that during the diastolic phase, blood pressure is produced by the force of the elastic walls of the arteries pushing on the blood to keep all the tubes filled. This pressure, indicated by the lower number of the blood pressure measurement, is called the *diastolic pressure*, the pressure in the circulation when the heart is filling up with your blood. If your blood pressure is 120 over 80, then the diastolic pressure is 80.

A blood pressure measurement always includes two numbers, the systolic pressure and the diastolic pressure. It was once thought that it was normal for the top number, the systolic pressure, to become higher as people grew older. Consequently, doctors believed that it was more important to keep the lower number, the diastolic number, within bounds. It is now known that *both numbers are equally important* to the preservation of your good health. Some physicians may still not be aware of this. It would be wise to find out if your own doctor has this knowledge. If either the top or the bottom number is elevated, you may require treatment.

When are these numbers elevated? We'll get to that later. First, it is important to establish the conditions which are required to ensure the accuracy of your blood pressure measurement. You certainly don't want an incorrect reading which falsely tells you that your pressure is elevated and commits you to unnecessary treatment for the rest of your life. Neither do you want to be told that your blood pressure is normal if it is in fact high.

3

ENSURING THE ACCURACY OF YOUR BLOOD PRESSURE MEASUREMENT

In the last chapter, you learned that systolic blood pressure is the pressure in your arteries when the heart is at the peak of its contraction, pushing the blood through your circulation, and that systolic blood pressure is measured by listening for the first sound made by the blood streaming through the narrow opening of the artery when the pressure in the blood pressure cuff is lowered just enough so that the artery goes from completely closed to almost completely closed. You also learned that the diastolic blood pressure, the pressure in your arteries when the heart is at rest, filling with blood, is caused by the elastic walls of the arteries pushing on the blood within them, and that the diastolic blood pressure is measured by listening for the last soft tapping sound which can be heard as the pressure in the blood pressure cuff is slowly released.

Accurate measure of blood pressure requires:

1. A blood pressure cuff which is the proper size for your arm and which is equipped with an accurate pressure gauge.

2. A stethoscope which is capable of properly amplifying the blood pressure sounds, and a quiet place in which to listen for these sounds.

3. Good hearing so that the soft sounds can be heard. Since the sound becomes softer and softer as the pressure in the blood pressure cuff is released, good hearing is especially important in determining the last sound, which reflects the diastolic pressure.

4. Adequate vision so that the numbers on the pressure gauge can be accurately recorded.

5. A careful and patient examiner who employs proper technique.

THE UNITS OF BLOOD PRESSURE MEASUREMENT

Before discussing each of the above requirements, a few moments should be spent explaining the units of blood pressure measurement. You have probably had your blood pressure measured, and you were probably told that the numbers are *something over something*, perhaps 120 over 80. What does this mean? One hundred and twenty what? As used here, that number is a measure of pressure—120 millimeters of mercury pressure. That doesn't help much, does it? Let's look at it another way:

When you fill up the tires of your car or bicycle with air, you have to set the pressure gauge of the air pump in order for the pump to deliver the recommended air pressure. For example, you may set the gauge at 28. The number 28 here is a shorthand way of saying 28 pounds of air pressure. The number 120 used in blood pressure measurement is the same sort of shorthand. But this time instead of pounds of air, we are talking about millimeters of mercury pressure.

Mercury is a liquid substance. It flows like water and can be used to create a simple blood pressure gauge which works as follows: A small open glass tube is placed upright in a container of the liquid mercury. The tube is arranged so that air pressure from the rubber balloon in the blood pressure cuff not only squeezes the arm but simultaneously pushes on the pool of mercury in the pressure gauge. As the pressure is raised in the cuff, it pushes some of the mercury up into the glass tube.

How far up does the column of mercury rise? One inch? Then the pressure in the blood pressure cuff is "one inch of mercury." One foot? Then the pressure in the cuff is "one foot of mercury." In measuring blood pressure, the metric system is used (10 millimeters is the same as one centimeter, or 0.4 inch). The length of the mercury column in the tube measured in millimeters becomes the blood pressure.

Mercury pressure gauges (mercury manometers) like the one described above are extremely accurate but are somewhat inconvenient. They are difficult to carry around because the mercury can spill out or the glass can break. Consequently, pressure-measuring devices have been designed which give pressure in millimeters of mercury but use springs or other kinds of pressure sensors. You may have had your blood pressure measured with one of these pressure gauges (aneroid manometers) as well. Usually the gauge has a round dial with numbers printed around the edge of its face. It looks something like the face of a clock, but it has only one hand instead of two. The hand rotates as the pressure changes, and the numbers on the dial reflect millimeters of mercury. The pressure gauge may fit onto the blood pressure cuff, may be held in the

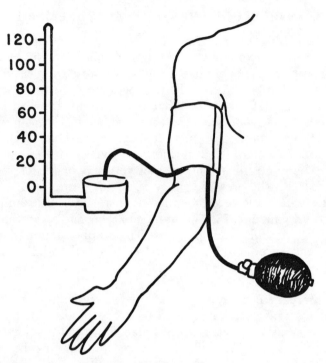

Mercury pressure gauge (Mercury manometer)

hand of the person measuring your pressure, or may be attached to the wall of the room in which you are being examined. If one of these gauges has been bumped around a lot or is very old, it may no longer be accurate. Every so often, the pressure reading of one of these dial-type gauges should be compared with the pressure reading of a standard mercury gauge to ensure that the readings are the same.

Something over something is usually written something/something. The slash is a shorthand way of saying "over." Thus 120 over 80 and 120/80 both mean the same thing: the systolic blood pressure is equivalent to 120 millimeters of mercury and the diastolic blood pressure is equivalent to 80 millimeters of mercury. Millimeters are usually abbreviated *mm*. Instead of spelling out mercury, its chemical symbol, *Hg*, is generally used. Thus 120/80 mm Hg is a shorthand way of saying 120 millimeters of mercury over 80 millimeters of mercury.

HOW TO ENSURE ACCURATE BLOOD PRESSURE MEASUREMENT

Now we are ready to discuss the five conditions cited above which must be met in order to ensure that your blood pressure is accurately measured. Unless proper precautions are taken, mistakes can occur. After this discussion, you will easily be able to evaluate whether the potential for error exists. If you think that there is a possibility that the person who measured your blood pressure made a mistake, *don't be timid*. Mention your concern and point out what you feel the problem may be. It is your body, and you have a perfect right to question the doctor, the nurse, or anyone else whose competency (or lack of it) can affect your health.

1. Essential: A Blood Pressure Cuff Which Is the Proper Size for Your Arm and Which Is Equipped With an Accurate Pressure Gauge

Let's review the steps that are involved in measuring your blood pressure. A blood pressure cuff is wrapped around your upper arm. Air is pumped into the cuff, squeezing your arm tighter and tighter until the flow of blood in the artery which brings blood to the arm has been stopped. Then the pressure is slowly released while the examiner listens over the brachial artery with an amplifying device.

Can you see how falsely high numbers can be obtained for the blood pressure? The purpose of the blood pressure cuff is to squeeze the artery beneath it. It is assumed that the pressure applied to your arm is the *same* pressure that is applied to the artery within your arm. It is assumed that the tissues lying between the blood pressure cuff and the artery have a lot of "give" so that the pressure in the cuff is transmitted fully to the artery. The tissues are thought to be like a highly flexible spring. When you push on one end of the spring, under normal circumstances, all the pressure is transmitted to the other end of the spring. If your arm is not too large, this method works. If you are not an unusually tall person, or if your upper arm does not have too much fatty tissue or too much bulky muscle, then the pressure in the standard blood pressure cuff will accurately reflect the pressure that is squeezing the artery. However, if you have either a lot of fatty tissue or very big muscles (or both), or just a very large arm, then the tissues of your arm do not work as a highly flexible spring. It takes more pressure to squeeze excess tissue. Not all the pressure in the standard blood pressure cuff is transmitted to the artery; some gets taken up by the excess tissues. In a case like this, your blood pressure will be incorrectly measured *if the standard blood pressure cuff is used*. Both numbers of the blood pressure reading will be falsely high. You will be told you have high blood pressure when your blood pressure may, in fact, be absolutely normal.

This error is rather common. For example, a very athletic 20-year-old man may have an extremely muscular upper arm. He looks healthy, feels healthy, and, in fact, *is* healthy. His blood pressure is entirely normal. However, he has the misfortune to have it measured with a standard blood-pressure cuff, and he is told that he has high blood pressure. This happens because the young man's strong muscles resist the squeezing action of the blood pressure cuff. The air pressure has to be pumped up relatively high just to get his tissues to squeeze in on the artery. The tissues in his muscular arm act like a very stiff spring. Although much of the air pressure pumped into the cuff serves only to overcome the resistance of his big arm muscles, it shows up on the pressure gauge as "blood pressure." There is no way of telling how much of the pressure recorded on the gauge is truly necessary to squeeze the artery and how much of the pressure only serves to overcome the resistance of the tissues.

If you happen to have an unusually large upper arm, you may well be told that you suffer from high blood pressure when you actually have a normal blood pressure. The standard blood pressure cuff is designed for the "standard" arm. If you are taller than the average person or have unusually well-developed upper arm muscles or have excessive fatty tissue deposited in your upper arm, you may not have an upper arm of average size. Should your upper arm be larger than normal, watch out! The standard blood pressure cuff may not work on your arm; the readings may be much too high.

This brings us to the question of cuff size. Think a minute. Try to remember the place in your doctor's office where your blood pressure is measured. Are all of the blood pressure cuffs identical or is there at least one cuff which is both longer and wider than the others? When your doctor measures your blood pressure there should be two or more cuffs to choose from. There should be at least one small (standard) cuff and one large cuff.

If you have been told that you have high blood pressure, did the person who measured your blood pressure take the pressure a second time with a larger cuff to make certain that the reading was correct? If there is a possibility that you have the kind of arm that is unusually large because it has either too much muscle or too much fat or because you just happen to be larger than the average person, then your reading should have been checked with a larger blood pressure cuff to be certain that you really do have high blood pressure and not just excess tissue.

The smaller cuff is the one commonly used to measure an adult blood pressure. (As we shall see in Chapter 13, still smaller cuffs are required to measure the blood pressure of infants and children.) There are two larger cuffs generally available: one is called the "large adult cuff," and the other, still larger one is called the "thigh cuff," originally designed to measure blood pressure in the leg. Both are longer and wider than the regular cuff, and one or the other should always be used if there is any question about the size of the upper arm.

The larger cuffs are designed to overcome the resistance of excessive tissue. To understand how they work we must return to the explanation of the units of pressure measurement presented earlier in the chapter. You learned there that the air pressure in a bicycle or an automobile tire is expressed as "pounds of air" and that the pressure in a blood pressure cuff is expressed as "millimeters of mercury." These measurement terms are actually shorthand for "pounds of air pressure per square inch" (also written "psi") and "millimeters of mercury pressure per square millimeter." The following explanation of the meaning of these units of area should help you understand how a large cuff overcomes the resistance of excessive tissue.

Consider an automobile tire. Automobiles come in various sizes, and large automobiles weigh more than small automobiles. A small automobile only requires a small tire to bear its weight. As we choose larger and larger cars, we also choose larger and larger tires. We do not use the same size tire for all cars, and we attempt to have the tire support the weight of the car by the tire's air pressure. We choose the right size tire for the right size car, and we maintain the air pressure about the same for all the tires. *Pounds of air pressure per square inch stay the same, but there are more square inches.* The same is true of blood pressure cuffs. When it is desired to compress the tissues of a large arm rather than a small arm, we do not try to overcome the added resistance of the extra tissue of the large arm by raising the air pressure in the cuff. Instead, we increase the size of the cuff. This way, we are able to overcome the resistance of the extra tissue without added pressure, just as we are able to overcome the extra weight of a larger car and keep the air pressure the same by increasing the size of the tire. By choosing a larger cuff, we apply the same pressure to a larger area of the arm. All the air pressure which is pumped into the cuff can be used to squeeze the artery; none has to be "wasted" to overcome tissue resistance. Now you have some idea of how size (area) overcomes resistance.

There is no mystery or guessing involved in selecting the right cuff for your arm. Rules exist to guide the person who measures your blood pressure. If there is any doubt which cuff should be used, the circumference of your arm can be measured with a tape measure. If the distance around the middle of your upper arm is more than about 33 centimeters (13 inches), then your pressure should be rechecked using a large cuff. However, it is seldom necessary to go to the trouble of actually taking measurements. Your doctor can usually decide which cuff to use simply by looking at your arm. *If there is any doubt about the size of your upper arm, then the blood pressure should always be checked with a larger cuff.* Incorrect cuff size is one common error in blood pressure measurement that you can easily prevent.

Although you can easily recognize the different sizes of blood pressure cuffs, it's not so easy to recognize when a blood pressure gauge is no longer accurate. It will require a combination of faith and judgment on your part. Here is a simple rule that might help: If the person who measures your blood pressure has taken the necessary precaution always to have at least two of the correct sizes of cuffs available, then probably attention has also been given to ensuring that the gauges are accurate. The standard is the liquid mercury gauge. This gauge does not lose its accuracy as it gets older or is moved about, although the glass parts should be clean and free from dust. The pressure gauges that look like clocks can become inaccurate. Every so often, they should be checked with a mercury gauge. If the gauge seems old, if it looks dirty, or if the glass protecting the face of the dial is cracked or missing, then the gauge may give a reading that is either too high or too low.

Since electronic blood pressure machines utilize arm cuffs, they are subject to the same mistakes mentioned above. Are you sure that the arm cuff of any such machine you might be using has been designed so that it will automatically adjust itself to the size of your arm? Again, if you have a large upper arm, it is quite possible that the automatic machine will give you numbers which are too high.

Remember, as well, that electronic blood pressure equipment must be checked frequently to be sure that accuracy is retained. This is a major objection to the electronic blood pressure machines which are located in such places as supermarkets, drugstores, and banks. They are most likely accurate when they are installed but it is rather expensive to maintain electronic equipment. Is anyone making sure that the machines are checked frequently to ensure that they remain in perfect working condition?

A final factor to consider when using electronic blood pressure equipment is the placement of the sound amplifier, which in this type of measuring device will be a microphone built permanently into the cuff. When the cuff is placed around the arm, you must be certain that the microphone is positioned so that it lies almost directly above the brachial artery. The design of the cuff and the design of the arm must match, and this is not always the case. If the microphone is lying too far from the artery, the first sound will be missed and the systolic pressure reading will be falsely low. Similarly, the last sound will not be detected so the diastolic reading will be falsely high.

In the final analysis, whatever the equipment used, the

only way you can protect yourself from inaccurate blood pressure readings is to be certain to have your blood pressure measured by someone you trust. If you have any doubt about the accuracy of the equipment, have your blood pressure checked again by someone else using different equipment.

2. Essential: A Stethoscope Which Is Capable of Properly Amplifying the Blood Pressure Sounds, and a Quiet Place in Which to Listen for These Sounds

Most of the stethoscopes available today will ensure adequate amplification of sound. It is unlikely that a stethoscope will be faulty. However, even with the best stethoscopes, the tapping sounds made by the blood are soft. This is particularly true as the lower number, the diastolic blood pressure, is approached. If the room in which your blood pressure is measured is noisy, it may be difficult for the examiner to hear the last sounds. Loud voices or music, the noise of automobile traffic, or the sound of a plane overhead can all interfere with the examiner's ability to measure your blood pressure accurately. Consequently, you should insist that your blood pressure be measured in a quiet place. A supermarket or shopping center or a drugstore may not be a favorable setting.

3. Essential: Good Hearing So That the Soft Sounds Can Be Heard

The hearing of an older person may not be as good as the hearing of a younger person. Doctors, like everyone else, are subject to the loss of hearing that age or disease may bring. There are specially designed electronic stethoscopes on the market which amplify sound. If the person who measures your blood pressure appears to have suffered some loss of hearing, a special electronic stethoscope or one of the electronic blood pressure devices should be used.

4. Essential: Adequate Vision So That the Numbers on the Pressure Gauge Can Be Accurately Recorded

Both the eyes and the ears are used to measure blood pressure. The eyes watch the blood pressure gauge while the ears listen to the tapping sounds made by the blood flowing in the artery. The eyes record the reading when the first and last sounds are heard. It is unlikely that faulty vision would falsify a blood pressure reading, but this possibility should be kept in mind.

5. Essential: A Careful and Patient Examiner Who Employs Proper Technique

The person measuring your blood pressure should have all of the correct equipment, but this will not be enough. Correct technique is also necessary. The cuff must be placed on your arm so that the rubber bag in the cuff lies above the artery. If the examiner has never measured your blood pressure before, the pressure should be measured in *both* arms. Once it is known which arm gives the highest reading, it is not necessary to continue this double measurement. The arm that gives the *higher reading is always the correct arm* to use for blood pressure measurement.

In most instances the right arm has a slightly higher reading than the left. Therefore this is the one that should be measured. The reason blood pressure is slightly different in the two arms has to do with the way the arteries are connected to each other. It is a simple matter of plumbing. Generally, the arteries which go out to the arms do not branch off from the central artery at the same angle. The artery to the left arm often has more pronounced angle than the artery which goes out to the right arm. Because the angle of the artery is more pronounced, the pressure of the blood flowing in the left artery tends to be a little lower than the pressure in the right artery. The artery with the higher pressure more accurately reflects the pressure in the main artery.

The person measuring your blood pressure must be sure that enough pressure is applied to squeeze the artery completely shut. This can be done by feeling your pulse while the pressure is raised. When the pressure is high enough, it will no longer be possible to feel the pulse. Care must be taken to lower the pressure in the cuff slowly enough to be certain that the first sound is really the first sound and that the last sound is really the last sound. If the pressure is dropped too rapidly, the examiner may go by the first sound, and you will be told that your systolic reading is lower than is really the case. If the examiner doesn't continue to lower the pressure very gradually and to listen patiently, the last sound may be missed, and you will be told that your diastolic blood pressure is higher than is really the case.

The position of your body may affect your blood pressure reading, but your blood pressure should stay in normal range whether you are lying, sitting, or standing. Unless you are taking medication, it is unlikely that your blood pressure will be markedly different in any of the three positions, and it is usually not necessary for the examiner to measure your blood pressure in all of them. It is *normal* for your blood pressure to go up when you exercise. Consequently, the person measuring your blood pressure should insist that you either sit or lie quietly for at least five minutes before the measuring process begins. After you have rested for five minutes, your blood pressure should be checked while you are either sitting or lying down. There are special circumstances when it is also necessary to measure your blood pressure while you are standing, and these will be described in Chapter 7 when medication is discussed.

If your blood pressure is found to be high, it should be checked three times. If two of the three readings are high, you may have high blood pressure. To be certain, your blood pressure should be checked again in a few days. If, again, two out of the three readings are high, then you do have high blood pressure, and you probably will need treatment.

If the blood pressure is *very* high in the first three readings (for example, a bottom number of 115 or greater), then there is no need to return in a few days for another measurement. A blood pressure this high requires further evaluation and treatment, and it is appropriate for your doctor to start tests and treatment immediately.

Now you know what blood pressure means, how it is measured, and how you can be sure that this measurement is accurately made. We will next discuss when blood pressure is considered to be high and how to determine when treatment is required.

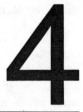

WHEN IS BLOOD PRESSURE TOO HIGH?

The best blood pressure is a low blood pressure. If there is sufficient pressure in your circulatory system to force blood to all parts
of your body at all times, whether you are sitting, standing, lying,
or moving from one position to another, why should the pressure
be higher? The heart is a pump, and every heartbeat is work for it.
Why make your heart work any harder than is absolutely necessary? The pump will last longer and function with the least complications if it does just the work necessary to get its job done and
no more. The arteries will last longer if they remain soft and flexible. If all your tissues are well nourished with blood, and if you
can change the position of your body rapidly without becoming
dizzy, feeling faint, or losing consciousness, then there is no need
for your blood pressure to go any higher.

If a blood pressure of 95 over 70 is sufficient to allow an
8-year-old child to be fully active and to live normally, is there
any advantage in a 40-year-old adult having a blood pressure of
120/80? Answer: No. If a 40-year-old adult can live normally with
a blood pressure of 95 over 70, then this is the better alternative.

Some adults do, in fact, have blood pressures of 95 over 70.
What does this then say about 120/80? Does it mean that the
adults with blood pressures of 120 over 80 suffer from high blood
pressure?

This is the dilemma with which your doctor is faced when
trying to answer the question: When is blood pressure too high?
One answer is that blood pressure is too high if it is *any* higher
than is just necessary to keep the body functioning well. However,
this answer is not of much practical use to you. What is needed is
to establish actual numbers which will serve as guidelines so that
both you and your physician can decide when your blood pressure
is so high that measures should be taken to lower it. The best way
to arrive at such numbers is to change the question. Instead of ask-

ing, "When is blood pressure too high?" a more practical approach is to ask: When is blood pressure so high that there is a definite risk that it may either shorten the life span or may cause an individual to suffer a stroke or disease of the heart, the kidneys, or the eyes? In other words, when is the blood pressure so high that treatment is clearly indicated? This question can be answered more satisfactorily and certainly more practically.

Certain guideline numbers have in fact been established. It is now known that any person 40 years old or less who has a systolic blood pressure of 140 millimeters of mercury or greater or a diastolic blood pressure of 90 mm Hg or greater has high blood pressure and requires treatment. (Remember that unless the numbers are very high, two out of three readings should be abnormal on two different days to establish that abnormality in fact exists.) Obviously, any numbers greater than 140 or greater than 90 make the need for treatment even more urgent. If a person is over 40 years of age, the numbers are raised to 160 for the systolic blood pressure and 95 for the diastolic blood pressure. Notice that only one of the two numbers which measures blood pressure has to be elevated to define high blood pressure. If *either* number is elevated, treatment is required.

Remember, these numbers are not exact. They are *guidelines* to help you and your doctor make decisions regarding your health. For example, a 42-year-old person with a systolic blood pressure of, say, 145 or a diastolic blood pressure of, say, 92, may require treatment. In what may appear to be borderline situations such as this, there are other factors known as "risk" factors which go into the decision whether or not to treat blood pressure. These will be discussed later in the chapter.

How were the pressures of 140, 160, 90 and 95 selected, and how was the age of 40 decided upon as a dividing line? The answers come in part from the life insurance companies. They make their money by betting on how long you will live. They long ago realized that the odds on living longer were much improved among those with low blood pressure—in fact, the lower the better. The life insurance companies asked the following type of question: Do men aged 35 with blood pressures of 142/90 live as long as men aged 35 who have blood pressures less than 142/90? It turns out that there is a tremendous difference in the life span of these two groups of 35-year-old men. The difference is so great, in fact, that one can say without hesitation that a 35-year-old male whose blood pressure is 142/90 has high blood pressure, and that it had better be treated properly or that man stands a good risk of either dying prematurely or suffering from a blood-pressure related disease such as stroke, heart disease, kidney failure, or damaged vision. This is why the life insurance companies will charge a man aged 35 with a blood pressure of 142/90 more money for life insurance than a man of the same age whose blood pressure is lower.

Long-term medical studies have also contributed to the establishment of guideline numbers for the treatment of high blood pressure. Medical scientists asked: Can we learn anything useful about the factors that control life span and disease through long-term observation of a large group of people all living or working in the same place? What can we learn, for example, if we study the population of an entire city or an entire company throughout the lifetime of the people who live in that city or work for that company? Such massive studies have indeed been accomplished, and out of them much important information has been obtained. For example:

1. High blood pressure is the single most important cause of strokes.

2. One-third of all heart disease is caused by high blood pressure.

3. The greater the blood pressure at any age, the greater the risk of death.

4. High blood pressure is a major cause of disease of the heart, brain, kidneys, and eyes.

Once medical scientists had identified certain diseases that unquestionably resulted, at least in part, from high blood pressure, they then tried to determine what blood pressure numbers at what ages clearly indicate a risk. We still do not have definite answers—studies in this area continue—but excellent guidelines did become evident as the scientists studied the data. These are the guidelines discussed earlier in the chapter. They can be summarized as follows:

● Any individual 40 years of age or less who has a systolic blood pressure of 140 or greater or a diastolic blood pressure of 90 or greater has high blood pressure and should be treated.

● Any individual over 40 years of age who has a systolic blood pressure of 160 or greater or a diastolic blood pressure of 95 or greater has high blood pressure and should be treated.

● Any individual over 40 years of age who has a systolic blood pressure within the range 140 to 159 or a diastolic blood pressure within the range 90 to 94 is in a borderline area. Other factors must be taken into consideration before a decision is made to begin treatment.

● High blood pressure should always be treated. You are never too young or too old to be treated if you have high blood pressure.

With the help of the above information amassed by insurance companies and medical scientists, we can arrive at a more satisfactory answer to the question: When is blood pressure too high? Blood pressure is too high if it increases the risk of early death or the development of severe, crippling disease. Using this answer, it turns out that in America alone, about 60 million people have blood pressures that are too high. This means that about 15 percent of all white Americans between the ages of 18 and 79 run a much greater risk of dying, or of being paralyzed by a stroke, or of being crippled by serious kidney, heart, or eye disease than do the rest of the white population. As grave as this situation is for white Americans, it is even worse for black Americans. For reasons as yet unknown, high blood pressure is almost twice as prevalent in blacks than whites. About 28 percent of all black Americans between the ages of 18 and 79 suffer from high blood pressure and are in danger of developing any of the serious health problems that high blood pressure causes.

These grim statistics are not unique to Americans. The World Health Organization has extensively surveyed individuals throughout the world, and the results of such studies clearly establish high blood pressure as a global problem affecting immense numbers of people of all races and nationalities.

Most people who have high blood pressure don't realize they have it. They usually feel well and function normally, at least for a while. But sooner or later high blood pressure will lead to disease or reduced life expectancy. When will this deterioration begin? In one year? In 10 years? In 20 years? In 30 years? The higher the measurement numbers, the greater the potential risk.

WHAT ABOUT THE BORDERLINE ZONE?

Does a person aged 42 with a blood pressure of 143 systolic have high blood pressure? The present scientific information does not clearly document that the risk of a shortened life span or serious disease is great enough to warrant treatment. That doesn't mean that it wouldn't be beneficial to lower the blood pressure to, say, 120 systolic. What it does mean is that scientists are unsure just *how much more beneficial* a blood pressure of 120 is than a blood pressure of 143 in this circumstance. If there were an easy, effective, safe treatment available that was free of all side effects, then the scientists would advise treatment. A judgment has to be made whether or not the advantages of treatment outweigh the possible disadvantages. In the borderline zone it is generally advised not to begin *major* treatment unless other adverse health conditions known as "risk factors" also exist. It is important for you to know what these risk factor conditions are in order to help your doctor evaluate whether treatment is necessary in this borderline area.

OTHER RISK FACTORS

We have seen that certain serious diseases can be caused by high blood pressure. Let's now take a look at the other health conditions that are risk factors for the development of these same diseases. Why do this? Because, if a person who has borderline blood pressure also has one of these other risk factors, then it is known that treating the blood pressure is indicated. In other words, if one of these other risk factors is also present, it takes blood pressure out of the borderline zone and into the danger zone.

The following health conditions may increase the risk of early death, strokes, heart disease, kidney disease, or eye disease. If any of them exists, a blood pressure reading of 140/90 is too high *no matter what the age of the individual*:

Diabetes mellitus (sugar diabetes)

Preexisting heart disease (such as angina pectoris, prior heart attack, evidence of an enlarged heart on X-ray or electrocardiogram, heart failure)

Obesity (the more overweight, the greater the risk)

Family background (if one parent is known to have high blood pressure, there is increased risk; the same is true if there is a strong family tendency toward the development of either early heart disease or strokes)

Cigarette smoking (increases the risk by a factor of about three)

High blood cholesterol (increases the risk about as much as does cigarette smoking)

Periodic readings of high blood pressure when young (this means that an occasional blood pressure reading was abnormal during the teenage years or early twenties even though most blood pressure readings were not elevated)

If any of these risk conditions coexist with a blood pressure that is in the borderline zone, then blood pressure should be treated. At the same time, any of these other risk factors should be corrected if possible. We will discuss this further when we get to the treatment sections (Chapters 7, 8, and 9), but clearly cigarette smoking and obesity should be corrected, and it may be possible to lower blood cholesterol. There isn't much that can be done about the other risk factors except to recognize that, because they exist, it is important to treat borderline high blood pressure. Again, the presence of any of these risk factors makes the treatment of definite high blood pressure all the more urgent.

RISK FACTORS ARE ADDITIVE

Risk factors are additive. For example, an individual who has a definite elevation of blood pressure may have twice as great a risk of dying from a heart attack as an individual of the same age who does not have high blood pressure. If such a hypertensive individual also smokes, the risk may be three times as great. If this individual is also overweight, the risk may be five times as great, and so on. This is another reason why it is important not only to treat blood pressure, but to eliminate as many of the other risk factors as possible.

A WORD OF ENCOURAGEMENT

Thus far, this chapter has been full of gloomy thoughts and dire predictions. The aim here is not to frighten or depress you, but to give you the facts and a set of guidelines. And there is good news to come.

In earlier chapters you learned what blood pressure means and how to make certain that your blood pressure is measured accurately. This chapter has explained how you and your doctor can decide whether or not your blood pressure should be treated. In reading it, you may have discovered that you fall into the category where treatment is clearly indicated. Has your doctor advised such treatment? If not, you should ask why. You now have enough knowledge to be an equal partner in making a vital decision concerning your well-being. *And this is the good news*: Blood pressure is generally quite easy to treat. In most cases, it can be brought back to normal with only a small amount of medication and with minimal side effects. And further good news is that treatment of high blood pressure works. The risk of developing stroke, heart disease, kidney disease, or eye disease can be significantly reduced once high blood pressure is brought back to normal. The earlier blood pressure is treated, the better the result, but treatment is effective at any stage of high blood pressure. No matter how young or how old you are, if you meet the conditions for treatment set forth in this chapter, you can expect to benefit from treatment, and in most cases you can expect that treatment to be easy to follow, uncomplicated, and highly successful.

Now you know when high blood pressure should be treated and why it should be treated. In later chapters you will learn what forms of therapy are most recommended, how such therapy works, what side effects to look for, and what precautions you should take if you are taking other medications, if you are pregnant, if you are breastfeeding, or if you have other health problems in addition to high blood pressure. However, before these topics are discussed, you need to know what questions your doctor should ask you, what kind of a physical examination you should receive, and what kinds of laboratory tests your doctor should perform before starting treatment. This information will be the subject of the next chapter.

5

WHAT YOUR DOCTOR MUST DO BEFORE TREATING YOUR HIGH BLOOD PRESSURE

You have been told that you have high blood pressure. You feel confident that the numbers are correct because you know that the proper equipment and the proper technique were used. You know that the blood pressure cuff was the proper size for your arm. Your blood pressure was measured in a quiet room after you had been sitting or lying quietly for at least five minutes. Your blood pressure was measured three times while you were being examined, and at least two of the three readings were high. Unless your initial blood pressure reading was very high, your doctor had you return a second time to recheck the numbers. If your blood pressure was measured by one of the electronic blood pressure machines, you had the readings confirmed by a competent physician or nurse. You did not rely upon a casual blood pressure reading taken in a noisy shopping center, supermarket, or drugstore. You know that you really do have high blood pressure because:

● You are 40 years of age or less and you have a systolic reading (top number) of 140 or greater *or* a diastolic reading (bottom number) of 90 or greater.

● You are over 40 years of age and you have a systolic reading of 160 or greater *or* a diastolic reading of 95 or greater.

● You are over 40 years of age and you have a systolic reading between 140 and 159 *or* a diastolic reading between 90 and 94, *and* you have another of the risk factors listed in Chapter 4.

WHY CERTAIN PROCEDURES ARE NECESSARY BEFORE TREATMENT BEGINS

Why is your blood pressure elevated? Are you a woman taking the contraceptive pill? Did you take a diet pill on the day that your blood pressure was measured? Diet pills and contraceptive pills are some of the medications that can elevate blood pressure. Your doctor must question you about these and other medicines. Certainly you don't want to be subjected to an extensive series of tests and start blood pressure treatment if all that is required is that you discontinue a medication! Do you have any complaints that might indicate that you already have a problem with your heart, circulation, or kidneys? Your doctor will want to question you about your present state of health in order to decide which blood pressure medicines are right for you. Have you had medical problems in the past or do medical problems exist in your family that may indicate that you have one or more risk factors? These and other questions are part of the extensive *medical interview* which your doctor must perform before starting treatments.

Are there special factors that might be causing your elevated pressure? Perhaps you are one of those rare adults who has what is called "surgically correctable hypertension." If so, an operation may solve your problem and medications will be unnecessary. By thoroughly examining you from head to toe, your doctor may find important clues which suggest that you do have one of these rare types of blood pressure elevation. Have you had high blood pressure for a long time, or is it something which developed only recently? Is there evidence that your elevated blood pressure has already affected one of your vital organs? Should your doctor begin treatment cautiously and slowly or is there evidence indicating that a vigorous and aggressive approach to blood pressure control is necessary? Your doctor can obtain answers to these and other important questions by performing a very thorough *physical examination*, and this must be done before starting treatment.

What other reasons could there be for elevated pressure? Are there aspects of your metabolism that are unusual? Are you the kind of person who is very sensitive to medicine, the kind of person who must receive even the most ordinary of blood pressure medicines in less than the usual dosage? Is there any evidence of heart strain or damage to the kidneys? The results of certain simple laboratory tests will help to answer these questions, and your doctor must perform a *basic laboratory examination* before starting treatment.

It is important to remember that before accepting any form of treatment for your high blood pressure, you must insist on undergoing the three procedures noted above: an extensive *medical interview*, a thorough *physical examination*, and a simple but essential *basic laboratory examination*. These three procedures are all part of your blood pressure evaluation. Each is essential, and each must be properly performed before you begin treatment.

Each of these three important parts of the blood pressure evaluation will be discussed in turn. First, however, you should know that the vast majority of adults have what is called *essential hypertension* or *primary hypertension*. The cause of this form of high blood pressure is not yet known, but it is thought to be caused by a combination of inherited factors and excessive salt in the diet. Essential hypertension is far and away the most common form of high blood pressure, and it is always treated medically, never surgically. Except in children, high blood pressure that can be corrected by surgical means is relatively rare.

Searching for a rare form of high blood pressure is only one of the reasons that your doctor must conduct a proper evaluation before beginning treatment. Some of the other reasons are even more important. You must receive the right medicine in the right dosage for the right reason. You must be protected from the adverse effects of medicines. You must be certain that one medication that you are taking will not be offset or be made more potent by another medication. You must be certain that *all* your health problems are treated and not just your high blood pressure. None of this can be accomplished unless you receive a full examination before treatment is started.

The following information is meaningful to all who have high blood pressure. If you are reading this book to help you to understand the blood pressure problems of an infant or youth, you will want to supplement this information with the information presented in Chapter 13.

THE MEDICAL INTERVIEW

Before performing any tests or prescribing any medications, your doctor should ask you many questions about your family, your past illnesses, your dietary and social habits, your present medications, and your present state of health. Your answers to these and other questions will provide information which is of vital importance. Simply by asking questions, your doctor may be able to discover the reason for your elevated blood pressure. It would be unwise and it could prove dangerous for your doctor to initiate therapy until this important part of your blood pressure evaluation is completed. The following are the areas your doctor must carefully investigate during the interview:

Your Family History In the last chapter you learned that a family tendency toward high blood pressure, early heart disease, or stroke is a definite risk factor. If you have a borderline blood pressure elevation, the decision to take medication may well rest upon information that you can supply about your own family. If either of your parents is known to have high blood pressure, to have early heart disease, or to have suffered an early stroke, then you have a risk factor which indicates that you should be treated. The greater the number of family members affected, the larger the risk.

Your Past Medical History Your doctor can obtain many important clues about the nature of your blood pressure problem by reviewing with you the nature of your past medical problems. In addition, this line of questioning may identify a risk factor that may be the deciding point in whether or not to treat a borderline blood pressure reading. As noted in the last chapter, even a single recording of an abnormally high blood pressure during your teenage years or early twenties indicates that you are at risk for developing a serious blood pressure problem. Your doctor needs to review the results of prior readings carefully with you. Perhaps your blood pressure was once measured as part of an evaluation for a college physical, for induction into the armed forces, during pregnancy, for life insurance purposes, or as part of a job physical examination.

It is important to remember that even a single abnormally high reading recorded in your past should never be dismissed as "just being too nervous." Not all people raise their blood pressure when they are nervous or anxious. Those who do may have a risk factor.

An inquiry into your medical past may also give clues about the cause of your blood pressure elevation. Did you have a kidney disease when you were a youth? Were you ever told that you had protein or blood in your urine? Did you ever suffer an accident which caused injury to the kidney? A yes answer to any of these questions may indicate that the source of your high blood pressure condition is underlying kidney disease.

It is also important to know when your blood pressure was last reported to be normal. If you are less than 25 or greater than 50 years of age and you know that within the past year your blood pressure was normal, this may indicate that your high blood pressure problem has developed rather suddenly. This is unusual. Most adults who develop high blood pressure do so between the ages of 25 to 50. Often, the numbers at first are mainly normal, then they fluctuate—sometimes normal, sometimes high—and then they become mainly elevated. Many adults begin by having what is called *labile* or fluctuating high blood pressure. If your blood pressure is suddenly found to be consistently high when you know that until quite recently it was consistently normal, this may be a clue that something new has happened to you and that you have one of the rarer kinds of blood pressure rather than the usual essential hypertension. This is especially true if you are less than 25 or more than 50 years old.

There are certain medications that definitely should be avoided and others that should be used with extreme caution if you have ever suffered from certain diseases. Some medications will aggravate conditions that presently exist. Some may even activate diseases that are no longer present. Your doctor must search into your past. Did you once have asthma? One common class of blood pressure medicines may activate latent asthma. Did you once have heart pain? Another medicine can bring out angina pectoris. Have you ever had trouble with your liver? With your kidneys? If so, some medicines should be used with caution, and others may require a reduced dosage.

Your Dietary Habits Consumption of too much salt is generally accepted to be a common predisposing factor to the development of high blood pressure. Often, high blood pressure can be reduced to normal levels merely by eliminating excess salt from the diet. Your doctor should review your food preferences with you and find out whether, either knowingly or unknowingly, you are eating a lot of salt. (Because salt is such an important issue, Chapter 8 will show you which types of food are excessively salty and how to plan a diet which is low in salt.) Did you know that eating too much licorice can cause high blood pressure? Not many people eat enough licorice to actually elevate their pressure, but there is an occasional person who is a real licorice lover. It would be a shame to start medication if all that is needed is to find yourself a new treat!

Foods which can raise your blood cholesterol will not raise your blood pressure. However, since the combination of high cholesterol and high blood pressure is three times as serious as high blood pressure alone, your doctor should review this aspect of your diet with you as well. You should find out whether you have a tendency to eat those foods which are known to contribute to high cholesterol. This way, your doctor can properly advise you how to make changes that will protect your blood cholesterol level.

Your Social Habits Alcohol in moderation is fine. No one has ever produced any evidence to suggest that a moderate amount of alcohol is detrimental to the health of an individual who has high blood pressure. This is also true of the other common social drinks: tea, coffee, and cocoa. Medical scientists have yet to produce any evidence to suggest that drinking tea, coffee, or cocoa are in any way hazardous to individuals with high blood pressure. *This is not the case with cigarette smoking!*

Cigarette smoking is a definite health hazard all on its own. The risk of premature death or of the development of a serious blood-pressure-related illness more than doubles if an individual who has high blood pressure also smokes cigarettes. Remember that smoking cigarettes is a risk factor. If your blood pressure falls within the borderline range and you smoke cigarettes, you should stop smoking and should begin blood pressure treatment. Cigarette smoking does not cause high blood pressure; rather, it is another factor which increases your risk of developing one of the serious conditions that can be caused by high blood pressure. You should not expect your blood pressure to return to normal levels just because you stop smoking, and even though you stop smoking, your blood pressure must still be treated. Your doctor must discuss your smoking habits with you and help you to stop.

Your Present Medications Certain medications commonly raise blood pressure. You are probably well aware that contraceptive pills and other medicines which contain female hormones may cause high blood pressure. Almost always, the blood pressure will return to normal once these medications are stopped, but it may take up to one year for this to happen. Your doctor needs to ask you about such medication. Treatment of your elevated pressure may require no more than stopping the pill. (Because the issue of the pill and other medicines which contain female hormones is so important, Chapters 10 and 11 are entirely devoted to this topic.) You may also be aware that diet pills may raise your blood pressure. Your doctor must inquire whether you have taken a diet pill within 24 hours of checking your blood pressure.

You may not be aware that common cold tablets, allergy preparations, and sinus preparations may temporarily raise the blood pressure. These medications can be obtained without prescription, and they are quite safe. Usually they contain two components, an antihistamine and a decongestant. The antihistamine helps to prevent allergic reactions from the dusts, molds, plant pollens, and insect hair that get into the air. The antihistamines are also mild and safe sedatives, and this slight sedative effect is often beneficial to one suffering an upper respiratory ailment or an eye irritation. The decongestant part of the preparation is the component that may temporarily raise blood pressure. Usually this decongestant is either ephedrine or pseudoephedrine. They work by constricting the small blood vessels in the mucous membranes of the upper airways and about the eyes. By shrinking the mucous membranes, they may relieve the discomfort of a stuffy nose or blocked ears or irritated eyes. Because it constricts the small blood vessels, a decongestant may temporarily raise blood pressure. Your doctor must inquire about your usage of this common type of medication. If you are told that you have high blood pressure, and if you have taken either a diet pill or one of the decongestant preparations within 24 hours of the blood pressure measurement, your doctor should instruct you to stop medication and return again in a few days for another blood pressure reading.

Medications may interact with each other. One medication may counteract the effect of another medication, or one medication may increase the potency of another. Your doctor must find out about *all* the medications you take. It may be necessary to avoid certain medication combinations. It may well be necessary to alter the dosage of certain medications. It is especially important for you to let your doctor know if you are taking heart medications, or if you are receiving any medications from a psychiatrist or a mental health clinic, or if you are taking medication to prevent or alleviate fluid retention. *Be certain to inform your doctor of all your medicines no matter how trivial they may seem to you.*

All the medicines commonly employed to treat high blood pressure will be discussed in Chapter 7. At that time, you will be told which other common medicines that you may be taking have the potential of significantly interacting with any of your blood pressure medicines. Fortunately, the important interactions are few, and it will not be difficult to be sure that you are protected in case your physician forgets to warn you.

Your Present State of Health It is important for your doctor to determine whether or not you have any complaints which may indicate that you have preexisting heart disease, kidney disease, or disease of the blood vessels. If any of these conditions already exist and you have high blood pressure, an aggressive approach to therapy may be indicated. Your doctor must also carefully inquire whether you have any complaints which suggest the presence of a condition that can be made worse by certain commonly used blood pressure medications. For example, do you have symptoms that suggest any form of lung disease? Some medicines can either aggravate or induce a breathing disorder. Do you have a tendency to depression? Certain medicines may make depression worse. What about dizzy spells? Some medicines may predispose you to dizzy spells. Your doctor must question you in all of these areas. Your doctor must ask you questions which will give important information about the function of your heart, your lungs, and all the other important organs.

THE PHYSICAL EXAMINATION

Your doctor must examine you thoroughly from head to toe. Certain parts of the physical examination take on a special importance when you are being evaluated for high blood pressure. Of course, your blood pressure itself must be measured correctly. How you can ensure that this is done has already been discussed at length. The easiest way to inform you of the especially important aspects of the physical examination is to start at the head and end at the feet.

Eyes The arteries and veins which supply the back of the eye can be seen by using a special instrument called an *opthalmoscope*. The opthalmoscope has a very strong light which is directed into the eye. Your doctor brings the light very close to your face so that the instrument almost touches your eye. This allows your doctor to see clearly the quality of your retinal blood vessels. Some of the questions that your doctor can answer by looking at these blood vessels are: Are they nice and smooth or are they narrowed and bent? Is there any indication that any blood vessels have been under such a high pressure that internal bleeding has occurred? The back of the eye is called the *fundus* of the eye, and this part of the physical examination is called an examination of the optic fundus or a fundoscopic examination.

Neck The large blood vessels which go up to the brain can be felt in the neck, and your doctor should gently press upon both sides of the neck in order to determine if there is a good full pulse in all the vessels. A weak pulse in *any* blood vessel might indicate a buildup of cholesterol. Obviously, knowledge of the quality of the blood vessels which bring blood to the brain is of extreme importance. If a blood vessel contains a cholesterol buildup, there may be some blockage to the blood flow. As the blood flows by the partially blocked area, it may make a rippling noise which your doctor can hear with the stethoscope. Thus, your doctor should also gently apply the stethoscope to both sides of the neck to determine if any unusual noises are present. The thyroid gland is also in the neck. Occasionally, an overactive thyroid can be a cause of increased blood pressure. Since an overactive thyroid gland is often enlarged, your doctor should gently feel the area of the thyroid to check for possible enlargement.

Chest Your doctor should carefully listen to your heart to determine the quality of the heart tones and to determine if there are any abnormal tones present. Once in a great while an individual is born with a partial narrowing of the large vessel (aorta) which carries blood immediately away from the heart and out into the circulation. In these rare cases the heart must work harder to force blood out into the circulation, and the blood pressure will be elevated. The doctor will be able to hear the noise made by the blood flowing past the narrowed section of the aorta. Other heart tones may help your doctor decide whether the heart has been working under a high pressure for some time and whether the muscles of the heart have become enlarged or strained.

Abdomen The large vessel (aorta) which carries blood away from the heart continues through the chest and into the abdomen. At the lower part of the abdomen it branches into two sections which supply the blood to the legs. In the upper part of the abdomen, two large blood vessels branch off the aorta to supply blood to the kidneys. By listening over this area of the abdomen with the stethoscope, your doctor may be able to hear noises which suggest that one of the arteries to the kidneys is partially blocked. In children and young adults, such a blockage may exist because of abnormal development of the blood supply to the kidneys. In older adults, a blockage here is usually the result of a buildup of cholesterol. By listening over the kidney areas, your doctor may find other clues to suggest that the blood supply to one or both kidneys is impaired. (In Chapter 9 you will learn later that this is one of the rare instances in which surgery is often a better method of treating high blood pressure than medication.)

If the kidneys are enlarged, your doctor may be able to feel them by pressing on the abdomen. Such enlargement is caused by a condition called *polycystic kidneys*. This is an inherited form of kidney disease and also causes high blood pressure. Fortunately, it is rare. Unfortunately, it cannot be corrected by surgery.

Legs Although the blood vessels which supply the arms seldom become blocked by cholesterol buildup, this is not true of the blood vessels which supply the legs. Your doctor can feel the quality of the arteries that supply blood to the legs at the groin, at the knees, and at the feet. A weak pulse in any of these areas may indicate a cholesterol buildup.

The aspects of the physical examination highlighted above concern the assessment of high blood pressure. However, the overall examination should be as thorough as possible so that your doctor can detect and correct *any other* health problem that you might also have.

THE BASIC LABORATORY EXAMINATION

The basic set of laboratory tests which your doctor should perform before starting treatment can all be performed in the office or clinic. Hospitalization is almost never required to evaluate an adult who has been discovered to have high blood pressure. Your doctor should hospitalize you only for very special reasons, and performing the basic required tests is *not* one of these reasons.

There are five reasons that tests are required before treatment of your blood pressure is begun:

1. *To look for other risk factors.* If other risk factors are discovered, then borderline high blood pressure should be treated. Your doctor should make every effort to correct these other risk factors at the same time that your blood pressure is treated. Diabetes mellitus (sugar diabetes) and a high cholesterol level are two risk factors which can be detected by the laboratory examination. Consequently, your doctor should have a sample of your blood checked for sugar and cholesterol.

2. *To look for underlying health conditions which may be either caused by high blood pressure or aggravated by high blood pressure.* An extremely high blood pressure or any elevation of blood pressure which has existed for a long time may cause either heart enlargement or heart strain. An electrocardiogram and a chest X-ray may detect either of these conditions. An electrocardiogram is a simple and entirely painless test which gives a picture of your heart function by measuring its electrical activity. An X-ray of your chest will allow your doctor to evaluate the size of your heart. Extremely high or prolonged high blood pressure can also cause damage to the kidneys. Your doctor may be able to tell whether such damage has occurred by examining a specimen of your urine (*urinalysis*). The kidneys function to clear the blood of wastes. If kidney function is reduced, your doctor can tell this by measuring either the BUN (blood urea nitrogen) or the creatinine level of your blood. The BUN and the creatinine are natural byproducts of tissue metabolism. They are removed from the tissues by the blood stream and taken to the kidneys where they are eliminated from the body by excretion into the urine. If kidney function is impaired, they will appear in the blood in higher than normal concentration. Usually both are checked, and all that is required is a small tube of blood. In fact, these blood chemicals can be checked by using the same sample taken to measure the cholesterol and the sugar.

3. *To determine if any of the blood pressure medications that you may need should be given in altered dosage.* One of the most important classes of blood pressure medications, the diuretics, act directly on the kidneys. Almost every person who requires medication for blood pressure will need a diuretic. Which diuretic will your doctor choose? To answer that question, your kidney function must be tested. This is done by measuring the level of your BUN or creatinine, or both (the same tests described above). A single measurement from a single tube of blood is all that is required.

4. *To look for one of the rare forms of high blood pressure,*

forms other than the common essential hypertension. Two rare hormonal abnormalities can cause high blood pressure: Cushing's disease and hyperaldosteronism. These will be explained in Chapter 6. A measure of the blood sugar and the blood potassium (K) will provide your doctor with information to suggest that one of these rare disturbances of hormone function might be present. Again these chemicals can be measured in the same tube of blood taken to measure your cholesterol, BUN, creatinine, and blood sugar.

5. *To obtain certain baseline numbers which reflect the overall function of your blood, your kidneys, and your chemical metabolism.* Medicines that are used to control blood pressure commonly produce alterations in your chemical metabolism. These alterations are due to the effect of the medicines and are not an indication that a disease is present. When medication is stopped, these abnormal chemical values return to normal. It is important for your doctor to know these numbers *before* you receive any medication. Otherwise, if one of these numbers is later measured and found to be abnormal, it will be difficult for your doctor to know whether the abnormality is simply the result of medication or due to an underlying disease.

There is another reason why your doctor must know these numbers before medication begins. At times, a medicine may alter some aspect of your bodily function in ways that are unexpected. The medicine may produce a toxic side effect, also called a toxic drug reaction. All during the time that you are under treatment with medication, your doctor will periodically take blood samples to ensure that none of these toxic reactions occurs. Again your doctor must know what the values of the tests are *before* treatment begins in order to know that a later detected altered value may be due to medication.

The two remaining laboratory tests you will undergo are aimed at obtaining baseline figures for your kidney and blood functions. (Your potassium, sugar, BUN, and creatinine values—also altered by blood pressure medication—will already have been established by the tests mentioned above.) The first of these final tests is a blood uric acid test. Diuretics often raise the level of the uric acid, and, if the uric acid level builds up too high in the bloodstream, an attack of gout may occur or kidney stones may form. This is why, before giving a diuretic, your doctor will wish to know your blood uric acid level. Fortunately, this can be determined from the same tube of blood as all the other chemicals, so you don't have to worry about becoming anemic!

The remaining test you will undergo results from the fact that rarely a blood pressure medication may affect your body's ability to produce either white or red blood cells. Your doctor will therefore want to assess your white and red blood cells by ordering a clinical blood count (CBC) or *hemogram*. This requires only a small amount of blood, but it must be placed in a separate tube. It cannot be determined from the same tube that is used to measure all of the other necessary blood tests.

As you can see, the basic laboratory examination is simple and brief. Only two small tubes of blood are required. One tube is used to measure your blood sugar, potassium, cholesterol, BUN, creatinine, and uric acid. The other tube is used to measure the level of your red and white blood cells. The chest X-ray and an electrocardiogram are painless tests that take only a few minutes to perform. Finally, an examination of a sample of your urine, a urinalysis, completes the basic set of tests.

Now you know what to expect from your doctor before *any therapy* is offered to you and before *any other laboratory tests* are suggested to you. A thorough evaluation of your blood pressure includes a medical interview, a physical examination, and completion of the basic set of laboratory tests. All this can usually be accomplished in one visit to the doctor. Your doctor does not have to wait until all the laboratory tests return before initiating therapy. It is perfectly safe and proper to begin medication once the medical interview and physical examination have been completed and the samples have been taken for the laboratory.

WHEN IS HOSPITALIZATION REQUIRED?

Hospitalization is never required for the routine evaluation and treatment of newly detected, uncomplicated high blood pressure. If the blood pressure is so high that it has caused heart failure or kidney failure, or if there is danger of an impending stroke, then your doctor will wish to hospitalize you immediately. It is up to you to have your blood pressure checked at regular intervals so that the need for emergency hospital care will never arise. High blood pressure is easy to detect and its measurement is painless, rapid, and simple. Once detected, high blood pressure is easy to evaluate, and treatment is almost always successful. With just a little effort on your part, you should be able to avoid the need ever to enter the hospital to have your blood pressure treated.

The performance of certain complicated and sophisticated laboratory tests does require hospitalization. If, after completing the full evaluation discussed above, your doctor detects evidence which suggests that you might be one of the unusual adults who has a form of blood pressure that is best treated with surgery rather than with medication, then it may be necessary to hospitalize you to perform certain tests. These tests will be described in Chapter 9, where the surgical treatment of high blood pressure is discussed.

WHEN ARE OTHER LABORATORY EXAMINATIONS REQUIRED?

There was a time when physicians routinely ordered kidney X-rays when evaluating blood pressure. This is now known to be unnecessary. Kidney X-rays seldom are required, and they should be obtained *only* when there is some reason to suspect that the blood supply to either one or both kidneys is partially blocked. If there is a partial blockage, strong evidence to suggest this will almost always come out of the thorough evaluation of blood pressure described above. Unless this three-part evaluation (medical interview, physical examination, basic laboratory examination) provides definite clues that your high blood pressure may be caused by a problem with the blood supply to your kidneys, you should not be subjected to an X-ray of the kidneys, which is called an *IVP* (*intravenous pyelogram*). If an IVP is indicated, it is not necessary to be hospitalized.

When should you undergo an IVP as part of your high blood pressure evaluation? Only when your doctor has found definite evidence that you may have a form of high blood pressure that can be corrected by operating on the blood supply to the kidneys. In fact, the only time laboratory tests other than those discussed above are required to evaluate blood pressure is when your doctor has found evidence which suggests that you may have one of the more unusual types of high blood pressure. The IVP and other laboratory examinations which are necessary to investigate the rarer types of high blood pressure will be discussed in Chapter 9, which deals with "surgically correctable hypertension."

6

HOW BLOOD PRESSURE IS CONTROLLED AND HOW BLOOD PRESSURE MEDICINES WORK

You should be convinced by now that if you really do have high blood pressure, you need treatment. You know how to protect yourself from improper diagnosis. You know when blood pressure numbers are considered too high and when treatment is necessary, and you know how insurance companies and medical scientists decided upon these numbers. You know when to insist upon treatment and when to question the need for treatment. You are familiar with the three essential parts of the medical evaluation of high blood pressure, and you know not to accept any medication or to submit to any complicated laboratory or X-ray procedures until your doctor has given you this evaluation. You know how to protect yourself in all of these important areas. Now you need to know how blood pressure medicines work so that you can be certain you receive *the best possible treatment with the fewest side effects and risks.*

In order to understand how blood pressure medicines and salt restriction work, you need to know how the blood pressure control system of your body functions. You will then be in a position to understand that there is a logical series of steps that your doctor should follow in treating your high blood pressure. You will know that some combinations of medicines are logical and others are not. You will be able to evaluate your own blood pressure treatment program and decide whether it is as good as it should be. You will be in a position to answer the question: What kind of treatment is best for me?

THE BLOOD PRESSURE CONTROL SYSTEM: THE MACHINES AND THE COMMUNICATION NETWORK

The blood pressure control system was briefly described in Chapter 1. We will now examine it in more detail. It is not complicated, and you will have no trouble understanding how it works.

The blood pressure control system is composed of three machines which can raise or lower blood pressure; they are the *heart*, the *kidneys*, and the *arteries*. Their actions are regulated by a communication network which can tell them what to do and which sees that they all work together smoothly to keep your blood pressure normal. *The nervous system* is one part of this communication network. The other part of the network, known as *direct control*, will be discussed later in the chapter. Before examining how the nervous system works in regulating the three blood pressure machines, let's take a brief look at these machines and the role that each plays in determining blood pressure.

THE BLOOD PRESSURE REGULATING MACHINES: HEART, KIDNEYS, ARTERIES

The *heart* is a pump. It can push on the blood with either more or less force. If it pushes with more force, blood pressure can go up. If it pushes with less force, blood pressure can go down.

The *kidneys* work to keep the blood in good condition. They regulate the concentration of important chemicals in the bloodstream. They also regulate the amount of fluid in the body; they do this either by retaining salt and water or by eliminating salt and water. When the kidneys retain salt and water, the volume of the fluid in the body goes up, and when they eliminate salt and water, the volume of fluid in the body goes down. By changing the volume of fluid in the body, the kidneys change the blood pressure. When they retain salt and water, the excess fluid goes into the tissues, and the tissues become stiffer. When the tissues are stiff, it is more work for the heart to push the blood through the arteries and out into the tissues, and thus blood pressure can go up. Conversely, when the kidneys eliminate salt and water, the amount of fluid in the body goes down, and the tissues become softer and more flexible. Since it is less work for the heart to pump blood through the arteries and out into the tissues, the blood pressure can go down.

The walls of the *arteries* are flexible; they contain elastic tissues and muscles. When the muscles in the walls of the arteries contract, the arteries press with more force upon the blood they contain, and this can make the blood pressure go up. Because the openings in the arteries are narrower when the muscles contract, the heart may have to pump with more force to push the blood through them, and this can also make the blood pressure go up. When the muscles in the walls of the arteries relax, the arteries press with less force upon the blood they contain, and this can cause the blood pressure to go down. Because the openings of the arteries are wider, the heart does not have to pump as forcefully to push the blood through, and this can also cause the blood pressure to go down.

These three blood pressure regulating machines work together to keep your blood pressure under control. If something happens to one machine to cause the blood pressure to rise, the other two machines can made adjustments to bring the blood pressure down again. For this interaction to occur, however, the body must have some way to tell the machines what to do and to coordinate their actions so that they all work together. One way this is accomplished is through the nervous system.

THE BLOOD PRESSURE COMMUNICATION NETWORK —PART I: THE NERVOUS SYSTEM

The body controls blood pressure by a communication network that is something like a telephone system. There is a central switchboard which is able to receive all the messages and know what is going on in all parts of the body at any time. This central switchboard is the nervous system. The brain and other vital centers of the nervous system can send out orders along the nerves to the blood pressure regulating machines. The nerves, acting like telephone wires, carry these orders to their destination. When an order gets to a blood pressure machine, it has to have a way to signal its arrival. This signal is the release of a chemical called norepinephrine. Upon its release, norepinephrine is picked up by receivers (called *receptors*) in the blood pressure machine, and the blood pressure machine immediately carries out the order it has received.

Norepinephrine is like the telephone bell. You know when there is a message on the telephone because the telephone bell rings. The blood pressure machines know when there is a message from the nervous system because the chemical signal, norepinephrine, is released. The receptors in the blood pressure machines which pick up the switchboard's message are like receivers. In order for the blood pressure machine to receive the chemical signal norepinephrine, these receivers must be on the hook. As with a telephone receiver, if the receptor is off the hook, the message will not go through, even though it has traveled down the wire.

Here is the way messages are sent and acted on:

● The nervous system sends out an order to the heart: "Raise the blood pressure." The message travels along the nervous system to the heart, and the chemical signal norepinephrine is released. This chemical signal goes to the special receivers in the heart, and the heart then raises the blood pressure by pumping more forcefully.

●The nervous system sends out an order to the kidneys: "Raise the blood pressure." The message goes along the nervous system to the kidneys, and the chemical signal norepinephrine is released. This chemical signal goes to the special receivers in the kidneys, and the kidneys then retain salt and water so that the total amount of fluid in the body is increased and blood pressure goes up.

●The nervous system sends an order to the arteries: "Raise the blood pressure." The message goes along the nervous system to the arteries, and the chemical signal norepinephrine is released. This chemical signal goes to the special receivers in the walls of the arteries, and the muscles in the walls of the arteries contract to make the blood pressure go up.

DESIGNING BLOOD PRESSURE MEDICINES

It may surprise you to know that you now have all the information you need in order to understand how *all* the blood pressure medicines work! Before going on to describe the remainder of the blood pressure control system, let's consider possible ways that blood pressure medicines might be designed in order to lower the blood pressure. Knowing what you now know about the way the blood pressure control system works, what would you want the medicines to do and how would you design them?

1. You could design medicines that *prevent* the message, "Raise the blood pressure," from getting out of the nervous system. These medicines would somehow alter the ability of the telephone wire to carry the message. If the message can't get out of the nervous system, the blood pressure machines will be unable to carry out the order. Many blood pressure medicines work this way.

2. You could design medicines that *prevent* the chemical signal released by the nervous system from getting to the special receivers in a blood pressure regulating machine. These medicines would serve to take the telephone receiver off the hook. If the special receptors in a blood pressure machine are unable to receive the chemical signal, the blood pressure machine will be unable to carry out the order, "Raise the blood pressure." There are a group of related blood pressure medicines which work this way.

3. You could design medicines that *force* the blood pressure regulating machine to carry out the medicines' orders even though the message from the nervous system gets through. These medicines would, in effect, take over the control of a blood pres-

sure machine. The most commonly used medication to control blood pressure works this way.

All the medicines which are used to treat high blood pressure work in one of the above three ways. Some work by interfering with the ability of the nervous system to get the message, "Raise the blood pressure," out of the nervous system. Some work by interfering with the ability of the blood pressure machines to receive the chemical signal that tells them the message, "Raise the blood pressure," has arrived. Some work by taking over control of the blood pressure machines so that even though the message arrives, the machines cannot obey the order because they are forced to follow the order of the medicines.

In Chapter 7 all the medicines commonly used to treat high blood pressure throughout the world will be explained, and you will be told which part of the blood pressure control system they change. You will also be told why some combinations of medicines are logical and why some combinations of medicines are not logical, and why certain medicines should be used before others. When you understand on what part of the system the medicines work, you will find it easy to understand the logical sequence in which blood pressure medicines should be used.

However, before continuing the discussion about medicines, it is necessary to complete the description of the blood pressure control system. Although you now have enough information to understand how all medicines work to control high blood pressure, you are not quite ready to understand why high blood pressure occurs. There are different kinds of high blood pressure problems. One form is extremely common; the others are not. The best way to understand why your blood pressure can become too high is to understand how the body normally keeps blood pressure under control. Then it will be easy to point out to you the different kinds of things that can go wrong with the normal system and cause high blood pressure.

Thus far, you know that there are three blood pressure regulating machines that make the blood pressure go up or down. Each of these machines can receive a message from the nervous system. The message goes along the nerves. When the message gets to a blood pressure machine, a chemical signal, norepinephrine, is released by the nervous system. This chemical signal lets a blood pressure machine know that a message has arrived. The chemical signal attaches itself to special receivers in a blood pressure machine, the receptors, and the machine immediately follows the orders of the message.

THE BLOOD PRESSURE COMMUNICATION NETWORK
—PART II: DIRECT CONTROL

Suppose something happened to a part of the nervous system? Suppose the nerves for some reason were not able to bring a message to the blood pressure machines? If the communication network consisted only of the nervous system, and if the nervous system somehow broke down, this could spell disaster. To be absolutely safe, the body does not rely *only* upon messages from the nervous system to tell the blood pressure machines what to do. The body also allows each blood pressure machine to make decisions independently. Each machine has a way of deciding by itself whether the blood pressure is too high or too low, and each machine can act on its own to make a change in the blood pressure should that seem necessary.

This is a protective mechanism for the body, but it is more than that. It is also a way for the body to achieve surer blood pressure control. Both systems work at the same time. This means there are more gears in the system, leading to smoother blood pressure control. You can think of the advantages of having two control systems in terms of taking water from a well. You drop the bucket down into the well and let it fill up with water. Then you raise up the bucket by pulling hand over hand on the rope. The bucket ascends with a jerking motion, and some of the water is likely to spill. If, instead of directly pulling on the rope, you attach the rope to a system of gears and then turn the gears with a handle, the bucket rises from the well smoothly and evenly. There is now less possibility of water spilling as the bucket ascends.

Unfortunately, in spite of its dual systems, the blood pressure communication network does not always work normally. In fact, millions of individuals throughout the world suffer from high blood pressure. Something has happened to some part of the blood pressure communication network which has caused the blood pressure to rise too high. If you have high blood pressure, then something has happened to some part of your blood pressure communication network. Let's take a look at what kind of thing this might be.

WHY HIGH BLOOD PRESSURE OCCURS

Almost everyone who suffers from high blood pressure has the kind that is called *essential hypertension* or *primary hypertension*. Since this is far and away the most common form of high blood pressure, this is the kind that will be discussed first.

Essential Hypertension: Salt-Related High Blood Pressure

Essential hypertension (primary hypertension) seems to be directly related to salt. Two conditions, both of them common, are thought to be required to produce essential hypertension: (1) an individual must have an inherited tendency to get this condition, and (2) an individual must eat salt. If an individual with an inherited tendency toward essential hypertension does not eat salt, blood pressure probably will not go up. If an individual has an inherited tendency to this condition and eats salt, blood pressure probably will go up. The more salt that is eaten, the higher the blood pressure can rise.

Not everyone who eats salt develops high blood pressure. Those who have an inherited tendency to develop high blood pressure are said to be *salt sensitive*. If you have high blood pressure, then you are probably salt sensitive. This is why your doctor asks you whether or not other members of your family have high blood pressure. If one or more does, you are considered to have a risk factor.

There are a few areas of the world where salt is either very hard to get or has not been introduced into the culture. These tend to be remote and rather primitive regions such as small villages in New Guinea and some of the Solomon Islands. In such communities, high blood pressure is extremely unusual. Fortunately or unfortunately, salt is relatively abundant throughout the world. In America about 15 percent of the adult population is estimated to have high blood pressure. In some of the islands of the Bahamas and in certain sections of Japan the people eat even more salt than is eaten in America, and high blood pressure is even more common. For example, in certain Japanese farming communities, 84 percent of the population has high blood pressure, and the leading cause of death is stroke.

Medical scientists do not fully understand why eating salt produces essential hypertension in those who have a predisposition for the disease. It is known that if an individual who develops essential hypertension eliminates salt from the diet before it is too late, the high blood pressure problem usually can be corrected without medication. However, if an individual continues to eat salt, a time eventually comes when the blood pressure tends to stay too high even though salt is eliminated from the diet.

Many theories have been put forth to explain why an excessive intake of salt can lead to the development of high blood pressure in genetically predisposed individuals. None provides a completely satisfactory explanation. Although the sequence of events which leads to the development of essential hypertension is not completely understood, it is generally agreed that the *first* important event is the accumulation of too much fluid in the circulation, which develops this way: An individual who is sensitive to salt eats salt. The kidneys try to get rid of the salt, but because of some inherited tendency, they cannot eliminate as much salt from the body as they should. Gradually, excess salt builds up in the body. Water always follows salt. When the kidneys eliminate salt, they also eliminate water, and when kidneys retain salt, they also retain water. Thus, when an individual accumulates excess salt in the body, excess water also accumulates. Gradually, the total volume of fluid in the circulation becomes larger than it should be.

When there is an excessive quantity of fluid in the circulation, the heart has to pump a larger volume of blood. (More blood comes into the chambers of the heart, so more blood must be pumped out of the chambers of the heart.) This tends to raise the blood pressure, because blood pressure tends to rise when the heart pumps a large volume of blood, and blood pressure tends to fall when the heart pumps a small volume of blood.

Now a *second* important event is thought to occur which results in an even further rise in blood pressure. Thus far we know that there is an excessive amount of fluid in the circulation, and that this excessive amount of fluid causes the heart to pump a larger volume of blood. This, in turn, results in an excessive circulation of blood into the tissues. The tissues sense that their blood flow is excessive, and they believe that this excessive flow is inappropriate. Consequently, they decide to take corrective action. The tissues decide to tell the heart to stop circulating so much blood, and they do this by raising the blood pressure. How do the tissues raise the blood pressure? They do this by telling the arteries which bring them blood to become narrower through contraction of the muscles of the arterial walls. Since it takes more pressure for the heart to force blood through narrow arteries than it does through wide arteries, blood pressure rises.

Are the tissues reacting inappropriately by causing the blood pressure to go up? Not necessarily. In the normal individual this is a corrective action which leads to reduction in an excessive circulation of blood. Look for example at what happens when you become frightened. With the onset of fear, your heart starts to beat forcefully and rapidly. This rapid heart action results in a sudden increase in the flow of blood into your tissues. Your tissues sense that their blood flow has become excessive, and they take corrective action by making their arteries narrower. This makes it necessary for the heart to push more forcefully on the blood stream if the circulation of blood into the tissues is to remain the same, and your blood pressure rises.

Now the interaction between blood pressure regulating machines mentioned earlier comes into play. You will remember that one of the basic mechanisms of blood pressure control is the ability of one blood pressure regulating machine to reduce blood pressure when another of the machines raises blood pressure.

Since the arteries have become narrowed, the heart must push on the blood with more force to keep the blood flowing into the tissues as rapidly as before. Is it necessary to maintain this speed of blood flow? Your heart decides that the lowering of your blood pressure is more important than maintaining such a high rate of flow of blood out into the tissues. This is exactly the message intended by the tissues. The heart reduces the speed and forcefulness of its contraction, the blood pressure comes down, and the excessive flow of circulation into the tissues is corrected. A series of continuing adjustments takes place, and the final result is that your heart stops pounding, your blood pressure returns to normal, and the arteries which bring blood into your tissues relax.

Unfortunately, the individual with essential hypertension is not normal. We are dealing here with an individual who for some inherited reason is unable to handle salt properly. The excessive blood flow into the tissues is not due to a fright reaction; it is due to too much fluid in the circulation. Consequently, the corrective action which the arteries take doesn't work. The arteries narrow and cause an initial elevation in blood pressure. They expect this to be temporary, because they expect the heart to respond by reducing the forcefulness of contraction so that their excessive circulation is corrected. However, the heart cannot respond in the expected way. It has no choice but to continue pumping back into the circulation the excessive fluid which it receives. Since the heart cannot take corrective action, the muscles within the walls of the arteries are unable to relax. In fact, thinking that somehow the heart did not receive their message, the arteries narrow even further, and this results in a further rise in blood pressure. Soon essential hypertension exists.

If the individual can stop eating salt in time, everything can reverse and go back to normal. As noted earlier, however, if this process goes on too long, something irreversible occurs, and even though the individual eventually gives up salt, the pressure remains set too high. Medical scientists do not yet fully understand why the pressure remains elevated, but it seems to have something to do with permanent changes that occur in the walls of the arteries.

Since you probably cannot develop essential hypertension unless you eat salt, your doctor will always advise you to cut down on your salt intake when you are found to have high blood pressure. Removing salt from your diet may be all that is necessary to correct the problem. Doesn't it make sense not to take a medicine if you don't really have to?

If your blood pressure doesn't completely come down to normal when you eliminate salt from your diet, your doctor may decide to give you a medicine that *forces* your kidneys to eliminate salt. Medicine of this type falls into the last category of the three possible designs for blood pressure medicines discussed earlier in the chapter. *Diuretics* force the kidney blood pressure regulating machine to eliminate salt. But remember, even if you take a diuretic, it is still necessary to limit your salt intake to some extent.

If you take a diuretic and continue to eat excessive salt, you are not being fair to your medicine. The medicine wants to help get rid of the salt already built up in the body, but if you continue to add salt to your diet, the medicine has difficulty doing its job. Instead of getting by with a mild diuretic that has few side effects, your doctor will need to use a strong diuretic with more side effects. Does it make any sense to use a strong medicine if a mild one will do the job?

OTHER CAUSES OF HIGH BLOOD PRESSURE

In order to understand the other causes of high blood pressure, let us briefly review the blood pressure control system. The blood pressure can be regulated in two ways: by messages which the nervous system sends to the blood pressure regulating machines, and by the independent action of each blood pressure machine. It is to the body's advantage to have this dual system of blood pressure control, but on occasion having multiple sites of control may be a *cause* of high blood pressure. For example, the heart may decide on its own to start pumping too forcefully. Or, the kidneys may decide for some reason to retain excess salt and water. Or, the arteries may decide for some reason to become too narrow. Or, the nervous system may decide to produce too much norepinephrine and constantly send the message, "Raise the blood pressure," to the blood pressure machines.

Since kidney disease is the second most common cause of high blood pressure in the adult population, let's consider kidney disease first.

High Blood Pressure Due to Kidney Disease

As we have seen, the most common type of adult high blood pressure is essential (primary) hypertension. This accounts for about 95 percent of all the cases of high blood pressure. The next most common cause of high blood pressure in adults is kidney disease. Although only about 5 percent of all adults who have high blood pressure have it because of kidney disease, this percentage of many million individuals represents a fairly large number.

You have two kidneys. Each is supplied by a large artery which brings the blood to the kidney to be filtered and purified. Suppose the artery to one of the kidneys becomes partially blocked. What happens? The kidney finds that it isn't receiving enough blood. It wonders why and decides that the reduced blood supply must be due to a change in the blood pressure. The kidney has no way of knowing that it is the *only* organ in the body that is not getting enough blood. It doesn't realize that all the other organs, including the other kidney, are fine. The kidney decides that the body is in trouble because the blood pressure has dropped too low, and it decides to do something about it. It decides it had better start the process of retaining salt and water to initiate the process which, as we saw earlier, brings the blood pressure up. Under some circumstances this would be exactly what the kidney should do; in fact such action could save your life. In this case, however, the kidney has made a mistake. It starts machinery going to raise your blood pressure. The kidney believes that it is making a low blood pressure normal again when in fact it is making a normal blood pressure too high.

To counteract the kidney's error, your nervous system sends messages to the kidney telling it to stop retaining salt and water, but the kidney, sure the blood pressure is too low because of the reduction in the blood it is receiving, keeps right on working to raise the blood pressure.

In cases where high blood pressure results from a partially blocked artery, the solution is to operate on the artery, *if this can be safely done*. When the blood supply to the kidney in question is improved, that kidney will cease its inappropriate activity and the pressure will fall to normal. If the narrowing of the artery can be corrected by an operation, the malfunction is called *surgically correctable hypertension*.

Usually, the blood supply to the kidney is reduced not because of a blockage in the large artery which brings the blood into that organ, but because the small arteries inside the kidney are damaged by some kind of kidney disease. Such disease might take the form of *nephritis*, or infection in the kidney causing scar formation, or it may be the result of one of the rare diseases that can damage the arteries within the kidney, such as *lupus erythematosis* or *scleroderma*. Whether the damage is to the large artery which brings blood to the kidney or whether the damage is within the kidney itself, the end result is the same. The kidney interprets the reduction in its flow of blood to mean "low blood pressure" and starts the process of raising the blood pressure. If the problem involves the blood supply within the kidneys, and it usually does, then surgery will not help. Fortunately, blood pressure medicine will bring the pressure down to normal.

It should be noted that the problems discussed above are not limited to one or the other kidney. They can occur to both kidneys at the same time and, in fact, often do.

How can your doctor tell if the large artery to the kidney is partially blocked so that surgery can be recommended? This will be explained in Chapter 9.

High Blood Pressure Due to Anxiety or Tension

What about chronic anxiety and tension? Individuals who have high blood pressure commonly blame it on their nerves. "Boy, I had a bad day at work, Doc. If you don't find my blood pressure elevated today, it never will be!" This reasoning is false. If two out of three blood pressure readings are elevated after five minutes of sitting or lying quietly on two different days, then almost certainly this person has true high blood pressure. Fright, anxiety, and tension may briefly raise the blood pressure, but most chronically anxious or tense individuals do *not* have high blood pressure. Those that do, need treatment and treatment is *not* sedatives or tranquilizers. Again, sedatives and tranquilizers are not part of the treatment of high blood pressure. The treatment of high blood pressure is salt restriction, weight loss, and, if necessary, blood pressure medication. Rarely, treatment requires surgery.

High Blood Pressure Due to Heart Disease or an Overactive Thyroid Gland

There are no diseases of the heart itself which cause high blood pressure. There are, however, certain conditions which cause the heart to pump too rapidly and too forcefully and thereby cause the blood pressure to rise. The most common of these conditions is fright. As noted above, an individual is suddenly frightened, the heart starts beating very swiftly and strongly, and this will briefly cause the blood pressure to rise. This is *not* a disease.

There seem to be occasional young people in their teens or twenties who have mild but true high blood pressure due to a heart which continues to beat too forcefully and too rapidly. This is probably due to a reason other than anxiety and tension. The treatment is not sedatives and not tranquilizers. Since the problem seems to be due to the too forceful pumping action of the heart, this is one of those rare instances when medication that works directly on the heart to reduce the forcefulness and rapidity of its pumping action can be helpful. You will learn about such medication when you read about the beta-blockers in Chapter 7.

Occasionally a person with an overactive thyroid gland will have high blood pressure. This has to do partly with the action of excess thyroid hormone on the heart. Excess thyroid hormone will speed up the heart's pumping action, and this in turn may lead to high blood pressure. In such cases, the proper treatment is to cure the overactive thyroid condition, not to administer high blood pressure medicines.

High Blood Pressure Due to Disease of the Arteries

Diseases of the arteries are rare and seldom cause high blood pressure. When they do, it is usually because there is damage to the arteries within the kidneys. This then sets off the process in the kidneys described earlier.

The walls of the arteries are flexible, containing elastic tissue and muscle. As individuals get older, it is normal for the arteries to become stiffer. The loss of elastic tissue is a normal part of the aging process, and thus it is normal for blood pressure to rise somewhat as individuals get older. A small rise in blood pressure as we grow older is considered to be an inevitable consequence of the aging process, and it is accepted as normal. But it is *not* normal for blood pressure numbers to go above the limits cited here. When blood pressure rises beyond these upper limits of normal, the aging process should not receive the blame. The major reason that blood pressure rises to abnormally high levels as we grow older is *not* the aging process: it is essential hypertension.

Diseases of the Nervous System Which Cause High Blood Pressure

To repeat, nervousness is *not* a cause of high blood pressure. Although many individuals tend to attribute their tendency to high blood pressure to anxiety or nervousness, they are mistaken. It is essential hypertension which is almost always responsible for their blood pressure elevation.

There is one rare condition of the nervous system that does cause high blood pressure. You will remember that the nervous system communicates with the blood pressure regulating machines by releasing the chemical signal norepinephrine. It is possible for an individual to develop a disease in which too much norepinephrine is continually produced. If this happens, high blood pressure results. This rare disease is called *pheochromocytoma*. It is treated by identifying the area of the nervous system which is making excessive norepinephrine and surgically removing it. Pheochromocytoma will be further discussed in Chapter 9.

High Blood Pressure Due to Obesity

Excess fat is a definite cause of high blood pressure, and it can be corrected by losing weight. The younger the age at which the excess weight is gained, the more likely it is that this weight will lead to high blood pressure. The more overweight an individual becomes, the higher the blood pressure may rise. The reason that obesity causes high blood pressure is not known. But given the documentation linking the two conditions, individuals who have high blood pressure should make every effort to lose weight.

Remember that overweight individuals should be certain their blood pressure is *correctly* measured. If you are overweight, you may have a large upper arm. If so, your blood pressure should be checked with one of the large cuffs as well as with the standard cuff. Chapter 3 explained in detail why this is so important.

Two Rare Hormonal Conditions That Cause High Blood Pressure
The adrenal glands normally produce a hormone called *hydrocortisone*. This is an essential hormone for normal body metabolism. On rare occasions, the body produces hydrocortisone in excess (*Cushing's disease*), and one of the effects of too much hydrocortisone is high blood pressure. Treatment of the condition often requires surgical removal of the gland that causes excess hydrocortisone production. Cushing's disease and its treatment will be discussed further in Chapter 9 where the surgically correctable forms of high blood pressure are examined.

Hydrocortisone in one of its many forms, and most frequently as prednisone, is one of the potent medicines commonly used by doctors to treat a variety of illnesses. If you are taking a form of hydrocortisone (often referred to simply as cortisone) and are told that you have high blood pressure, it may be possible to bring your pressure down to normal simply by reducing the amount of the medication that you are taking. The medicine may well be the cause of your blood pressure elevation.

The adrenal glands also produce a hormone called *aldosterone*. Like hydrocortisone, this is an essential hormone for normal body metabolism. As is the case with hydrocortisone, on rare occasions there is excess production of this hormone. One of the major effects of too much aldosterone (*hyperaldosteronism*) is high blood pressure. Here, too, the treatment may be surgical (see Chapter 9).

Now that you understand the blood pressure control system and the three ways that medicines can act upon the system to lower blood pressure, you are ready to learn about the medicines themselves. The next chapter will provide you with detailed information about every important blood pressure medicine in use today. At the same time it will show you the logic behind "stepwise" or progressive therapy and explain why this is the best and most effective way for treatment to proceed. It will not only enable you to ensure that you are taking your own medication in a way that is safe and relatively free from side effects, but it will also allow you to decide whether or not the particular medicine or combination of medicines that you are taking can reasonably be expected to give you the best possible result. If after reading Chapter 7 you should question your present therapy, you will be equipped with sufficient knowledge to discuss your concerns with your doctor so that together you can select a treatment program that will provide you with the best that modern medicine has to offer.

7

THE TREATMENT OF HIGH BLOOD PRESSURE WITH MEDICINES

In the last chapter you found out how the blood pressure control system works and learned about the mechanisms by which blood pressure medicines interfere with some part of the control system in order to lower the blood pressure. You also learned that there are three ways that a medicine can be designed in order to lower your blood pressure.

1. A medicine can interfere with the ability of the nervous system to get the message, "Raise the blood pressure," out to the blood pressure machines.

2. A medicine can interfere with the ability of a blood pressure machine to receive the message even though it gets out of the nervous system.

3. A medicine can force one of the blood pressure machines to obey its orders even though the message gets out of the nervous system and is received by the machine.

All three of these mechanisms are used in the treatment of high blood pressure. For example:

(1) The medicine methyldopa works by interrupting the message within the nervous system. Methyldopa interferes with the ability of the nervous system to get the message, "Raise the blood pressure," out to the blood pressure machines.

(2) The medicine propranolol works by preventing the chemical signal norepinephrine, which is released by the nervous system, from attaching to its receivers (receptors) in the heart and the kidneys, two of the blood pressure regulating machines. The organs of the body have many different receptors. Each receptor functions to allow a unique chemical messenger to make itself known. For example, when the pituitary gland (located in the brain) wishes to tell the adrenal gland (located in the abdomen) to

make more hydrocortisone, it does this by secreting a chemical messenger called ACTH into the blood stream. It is ACTH's job to go to the adrenal gland and give it the message "Synthesize more hydrocortisone." Since blood goes to all the organs, how is ACTH able to single out just the adrenal gland? The special receptor takes care of this. Only the adrenal gland has the proper receptor to receive ACTH. Consequently, although blood flows to all the organs, only the adrenal gland picks up the ACTH message. For blood pressure control, the receptor of interest is called the beta-receptor. This is the receptor which allows the norepinephrine message to make itself known. A beta-blocker medicine has the ability to prevent norepinephrine from attaching itself to the beta-receptor so that the message "Raise the blood pressure" cannot be delivered to the blood pressure regulating machines.

(3) The diuretic medicines lower blood pressure by forcing the kidneys to eliminate salt and water. They work directly on the kidneys, which are forced to carry out the orders of the diuretics even though the message from the nervous system gets through.

When your doctor decides that you require a medicine to treat your blood pressure, a choice has to be made. Which of these three mechanisms, each of which works on a different part of the blood control system, will be used?

Once this decision is made, another decision must follow. Which of the various medicines that work by the mechanism selected will be chosen to do the job? There are many different medicines that work by mechanism 1. Which is to be selected? There is a group of related medicines that work by mechanism 2. Which one of the group is to be selected? There are a number of medicines that work by mechanism 3. Which is to be selected?

Your doctor, then, has to make two basic decisions about blood pressure medicines. First, a decision has to be made about the method of attack, that is, which mechanism of interfering with the blood pressure control system will be employed. Once this decision has been made, your doctor must then decide which of the various medicines that have the desired unique mechanism of action will be chosen.

Does it seem complicated? Actually, it is relatively simple. There are straightforward guidelines which are used to select medicines. Following these guidelines makes the job of selecting medicines easy.

GUIDELINES EMPLOYED TO SELECT MEDICINES TO TREAT HIGH BLOOD PRESSURE

1. Your doctor will want to choose a medicine that will attack the basic cause of high blood pressure. Since essential hypertension is responsible for almost all of the blood pressure problems that phy-

sicians treat, a diuretic is often the first medicine selected *after* it has been determined that restricting the salt in the diet by itself does not completely bring the blood pressure down to normal. Remember that essential hypertension is thought to be caused by too much salt in the body. Diuretics work by making the kidneys eliminate excess salt. Diuretics attack the basic cause of the blood pressure problem.

2. Your doctor will want to choose medicines that will safely lower your blood pressure with as few side effects as possible. By thoroughly examining you before starting any treatment, your doctor will be able to reasonably predict the nature and the dosage of the medicines that should work best for you.

3. Your doctor will want to use as few medicines as possible. If it is possible to use only one medicine, then why use two? The fewer medicines that are used, the fewer the possible side effects.

4. Your doctor will want to prescribe medicines that are easy to take. It is easier to take a medicine once a day than twice a day. It is easier to take a medicine twice a day than three times a day. The more frequently a medicine has to be taken during the day, the easier it is for someone to forget to take it. This means that medicines which have a long duration of action are more desirable than those which will keep the pressure down only if taken frequently throughout the day. Of those that have this long duration of action, the long-acting diuretics and the beta-blockers tend to have the fewest side effects.

5. Your doctor will want to treat blood pressure in a *stepwise* fashion, that is, to start with the simplest form of treatment and progressively *add* treatment. The simplest treatment program is to restrict salt in the diet (and to lose weight). If this isn't totally successful, the next step is to add a diuretic or a beta-blocker. If this isn't totally successful, your doctor will want to add the next logical medicine. The salt restriction remains. The diuretic or beta-blocker remains. If it is necessary to add still a third medicine, the other medicines remain.

6. If blood pressure control does require more than one medicine, your doctor will want to choose combinations of medicines that employ *different* mechanisms of attack on the blood pressure control system. Since there are three mechanisms, each medicine selected should have a unique action. For example, if the first medicine chosen is a diuretic, which acts by forcing the kidney to eliminate excessive salt, then the next medicine chosen to use with the diuretic should be either a medicine that works by interfering with the ability of the message to get out of the nervous system (such as methyldopa), or a medicine that acts by preventing a blood pressure machine from receiving the signal (such as

propranolol), or a medicine that forces one of the *other* blood pressure machines to follow its orders (such as hydralazine, which works directly on the walls of the arteries, forcing them to become wider). There is only one relatively common situation where this guideline is not followed fairly strictly. It involves the medicines, like methyldopa, that interrupt the message within the nervous system. Other such medicines are clonidine, guanethidine and related compounds, prazosin, and the Rauwolfia compounds such as reserpine. Many of these medicines tend to have fairly significant side effects, such as making you sleepy or making you feel dizzy or lightheaded when you change position. The side effects can usually be controlled since they tend to be dosage-related: the smaller the quantity of medicine employed, the fewer the side effects. Consequently, even though they employ the same general mechanism, two of these medicines can be combined so that the dosage of each is kept small enough to reduce the possibility of your experiencing annoying side effects.

By following the above guidelines, it is possible for your doctor to create a treatment program that is logical and effective. If you are taking only one medicine, that medicine should almost always be either a diuretic or a beta-blocker. In the United States it is most common to use a diuretic first. Outside the United States a beta-blocker is often the first medicine chosen if the blood pressure elevation is only mild. Like diuretics, the beta-blockers tend to have few side effects, and many have a long enough duration of action to allow once a day administration. As long as the blood pressure elevation is mild, either a diuretic or a beta-blocker can be expected to control blood pressure. This is not true of the methyldopa type medicines. Methyldopa and the other medicines in this group all have the undesirable side effect of promoting fluid retention. As you know, fluid retention is a cause of high blood pressure. Unless they are given along with a diuretic, the medicines of this group lose their effectiveness. Their blood pressure lowering effect is soon neutralized by the gradual accumulation of fluid which they cause. In the individual with more severe high blood pressure, it is generally recommended that a diuretic be started before the beta-blocker is added. If you are taking more than one medicine, then *one* of the medicines is most often a diuretic. If you are taking more than one medicine, then each medicine should attack a different part of the blood pressure control system, except in the instances cited in guideline number 6. *Whether you are taking one medicine or many medicines, you should always limit the quantity of salt that you eat, and you should always lose weight if you are overweight.*

These guidelines really work. There is little mystery or magic to the treatment of blood pressure.

What do you need to know about the medicines that you are taking? You need to know by which mechanism they work on the blood pressure control system so that you can be sure that the choice of medicines is a logical one. You need to know the usual adult dosage. You need to know the common side effects so that you can be aware of what is happening to your body, and so you will know when to stop medicines if the side effects become too disturbing. You need to know what you can do to minimize the side effects of the medicines that you take. You need to know what other common medicines may interact with one of your blood pressure medicines and either make it too strong or make it ineffective. If you are either pregnant or nursing your baby, you need to know if a medicine will potentially harm the growing fetus or baby. You need to know if there are any medicines that you should avoid or use with great caution if you already have some other health condition or if some other health condition develops while you are taking a high blood pressure medication. Finally, you need to know if there are any specific instructions you should follow should you decide to stop taking one of your blood pressure medicines.

SIT BEFORE YOU STAND. STAND BEFORE YOU WALK

All medicines used to treat high blood pressure have a tendency to cause some lightheadedness or dizziness when you change position. For example, if you are lying down and suddenly sit up or stand up, you may feel as if you are going to faint. If you bend over and suddenly straighten up, the same thing can happen. This is to be expected, for what is the purpose of blood pressure in the first place? Its purpose is to ensure that all parts of your body receive an adequate blood flow at all times, no matter what your posture or body motion. Now what do blood pressure medicines do? They interfere with your blood pressure control system. When you take *any* medicine to treat high blood pressure, your blood pressure control system will be unable to respond to changes in posture as rapidly as it did before. This is why you are taking medicine! The fact that you experience a little lightheadedness or dizziness simply means that the medicine is doing its job. To prevent these feelings from becoming pronounced, follow this simple rule: *Sit before you stand. Stand before you walk.* This will give your blood pressure control system time to adjust.

DEHYDRATION

The symptoms of lightheadedness or dizziness will be much more pronounced if you become dehydrated. If you become sufficiently dehydrated, you might even faint when you stand up. This happens because the medicine has already made the blood pressure control system sluggish; if you are dehydrated as well, there is less blood to be moved where it has to go. Consequently, it is always important that you *avoid dehydration* when you take medicines to treat high blood pressure. Heavy sweating on a hot day can cause dehydration. Heavy sweating because of prolonged strenuous physical work can cause dehydration. Prolonged or uncontrolled vomiting or diarrhea almost always causes dehydration. If you do become dehydrated for any reason, you should do the following: (1) lie down as much as possible; (2) correct the cause of your dehydration; (3) temporarily stop your medicines until you can speak with your doctor; and (4) drink some liquid. The liquid you drink to correct your dehydration should contain salt if you have been either vomiting or have had diarrhea. You cannot safely correct dehydration by drinking water alone in these circumstances. Good sources of salty solutions are bouillon cubes and canned soups. This is one of those times when chicken soup really works! Generally, two or three cups of bouillon or a salty soup will correct your tendency to faint if you have lost fluids due to either vomiting or diarrhea.

GENERIC VS. BRAND NAME

All medicines have two (or more) names: a generic or chemical name and brand name. Some medicines are manufactured by more than one pharmaceutical firm, and each firm gives the medicine its own brand name. For example, hydrochlorothiazide is the generic name for a commonly used diuretic. This diuretic is manufactured by many different firms, and each calls the medicine something different. For example, there is hydrochlorothiazide (Hydro-DIURIL), hydrochlorothiazide (Hydro-Z-50), hydrochlorothiazide (Oretic), and hydrochlorothiazide (Esidrix). All four medicines named in the parentheses are identical; all are brand names for the generic medicine hydrochlorothiazide.

International Medicine Index While there are actually a relatively small number of medicines that are employed in the treatment of high blood pressure, there are a multitude of trade names, because many different pharmaceutical firms manufacture the same medicine, each under a different trade name. The International Medicine Index (page 247) will allow you to identify high blood pressure medications wherever you may be. It also gives the page numbers for the "potassium-sparing agents" and potassium supplements which are described in Chapter 8.

Medicines that are used throughout the world are included

on this list, although not all the medicines are available in every country. For example, many medicines are not available in the United States either because the manufacturers have not requested approval of the Federal Drug Administration or because such approval is still pending. The fact that a medicine is not available in one country but is available in another should not be taken to indicate that there might be something wrong with the medicine. Complex licensing regulations as well as marketing decisions of the pharmaceutical firms influence what medicine will be sold where.

BLOOD PRESSURE MEDICINE GROUPED ACCORDING TO THEIR UNIQUE MECHANISM OF ACTION

Medicines That Interrupt the Message in the Nervous System:
clonidine (Caprysin, Catapres, Catapresan, Catapressan, Clonilum, Clonisin, Dixarit, Haemiton, Hyposyn, Ipotensium, Isogluaron. Namestin)

guanethidine and related compounds (There are many. Ismelin is the most frequently used. Their chemical and trade names are listed on page 64.)

methyldopa (Aldomet, Aldomet-M, Aldometil, Aldomine, Dopalin, Hyperpax, Medomet, Methoplain, Presinol, Sembrina)

prazosin (Hypovase, Minipres, Sinetens)

Rauwolfia compounds (There are many. Of these, reserpine is the most frequently used. Their chemical and trade names are listed on page 68.)

Medicines That Prevent a Blood Pressure Machine From Receiving a Signal:
beta-blockers (There are many. Propranolol is the most frequently used. Their chemical and trade names are listed on page 72.)

Medicines That Take Over the Control of a Blood Pressure Machine:
diuretics (There are many. They differ in their strength and duration of action. Their chemical and trade names are listed on page 79.)

hydralazine—(also spelled hydrallazine) (Aprelazine, Apresoline, Apressoline, Dralzine, Hydralyn, Hyperazine, Lopress, Rolazine) and *dihydrallazine* (Nepresol, Nepresoline, Nepressol, Pressaline)

minoxidil (Loniten)

calcium antagonists (This is a relatively new group of medicines which have mainly been employed for the relief of angina pectoris but which are now also being used to treat high blood pressure.)

The dosages listed for each of the medicines below should be considered only as guidelines. Some individuals are very sensitive to a medicine and will require a smaller dosage than that listed. Others will be resistant to a medicine and may require a quantity much higher than that listed. You probably have no need for concern if the dosage of any of your medicines is different from that listed, but it will do no harm to discuss this with your doctor. In general, to find the dosage of medicine which is best for you, your doctor should start with a low dosage and gradually increase the amount of medicine over a period of days or weeks. The longer the medicine stays in your system, the more slowly the dosage should be changed. In other words, the dosage of a long-acting medicine should be increased more slowly than the dosage of a short-acting medicine. The goal is good control of your blood pressure with a minimum of side effects.

MEDICINES THAT INTERRUPT THE MESSAGE IN THE NERVOUS SYSTEM

General Remarks: All medications in this group tend to have prominent side effects of dry mouth and drowsiness or fatigue. Since the side effects of medicines are dosage related, it may be possible, as noted above, to reduce the side effects by using two of these medicines together, each at a lower dosage than would be used if either medicine was taken alone. A diuretic and salt restriction should almost always be used with any of the medicines.

Clonidine

clonidine (Caprysin, Catapres, Catapresan, Catapressan, Clonilum, Clonisin, Dixarit, Haemiton, Hyposyn, Ipotensium, Isogluaron, Namestin) Comes in 0.1 mg, 0.15 mg, 0.2 mg, and 0.3 mg tablets. The initial dosage is 0.1 mg twice a day. The usual dosage is 0.1 to 0.3 mg twice a day. The most common side effects are dry mouth and drowsiness or fatigue. Sexual impotence and dizziness are less frequent side effects. Usually these side effects disappear after you get used to the medicine. This can take up to one month. Salt and water retention are prominent, and a diuretic should always be taken with clonidine. *Important drug interactions:* The effect of clonidine may be reduced when tricyclic antidepressant medicines are also used. If you are being treated for depression, anxiety, or nervousness, you may be taking one of the tricyclic antidepressants. You will find the names of all the commonly used tricyclic antidepressants on page 238. If you are taking clonidine, and a tricyclic antidepressant is added to your treatment program, you must have your blood pressure checked to be sure that it does not go up. Your blood pressure must also be checked if a beta-blocker is added while you are taking clonidine, because the two medicines may work against each other so that their effectiveness is reduced. *WARNING:* Clonidine should never be stopped rapidly or suddenly. The dosage should gradually be reduced over about a two-week period. If clonidine is stopped suddenly, it can cause a severe and dangerous rise in blood pressure. *Pregnancy:* Not proven to be safe. Do not use. *Breastfeeding:* Not known if it appears in breast milk. Do not use.

The Guanethidine Group
This group consists of a number of chemically similar medicines. They differ mainly in their duration of action. Guanethidine (Ismelin) is the best known and most widely used of the group, and all the others are compared to guanethidine. The following table will allow you to identify which of the group you may be taking:

TRADE NAME OF MEDICINES OF THE GUANETHIDINE GROUP FOLLOWED BY GENERIC (CHEMICAL) NAME

Anorel • guandrel	Esbaloid • bethanidine
Antipres • guanethidine	Esbatal • bethanidine
Banthid • bethanidine	Hylorel • guandrel
Declinax • debrisoquine	Ismelin • guanethidine
Envacar • guanoxan	Tenathan • bethanidine
Esbalid • bethanidine	Vatensol • guanochlor

---

guanethidine (Antipres, Ismelin) Comes in 10 mg and 25 mg tablets. It is very potent and has a long duration of action. The initial dosage should be 10 mg or less taken once daily. Because the drug stays in the body a long time, the dosage should be increased by only about 10 mg a week. The usual dosage is 10 to 50 mg taken once a day. The most common side effects are lightheadedness and dizziness when changing posture or when exercising vigorously. Lightheadedness and dizziness may also occur after drinking alcohol or upon exposure to a hot environment such as a steam bath or very hot shower. It is essential that your doctor check both your *standing* and your lying blood pressure. It is common for guanethidine to produce a normal blood pressure while you are lying down but to cause the pressure to fall dangerously low when you stand up or when you exercise. It is very common for guanethidine to cause lightheadedness when you first get out of bed, and you should be especially careful to change position slowly when you first awaken. Diarrhea frequently occurs. If diarrhea cannot be stopped by reducing the dosage of guanethidine, you should stop the medication until you can speak with your doctor. Men may experience an inability to have an erection or an inability to ejaculate. This goes away when the medicine is stopped. Nasal stuffiness is a less frequent side effect. *Important drug interactions*: Numerous medicines used in the treatment of anxiety, depression, and other nervous disorders can interact with guanethidine to make it less effective. The same is true of some medicines that are used to treat nausea or dizziness. If you are taking guanethidine and one of these medicines is added to your program, you must have your blood pressure checked to make sure it does not go up. There are three groups of medicines that can do this: the tricyclic antidepressants; the phenothiazines (major tranquilizers); and the monoamine oxidase inhibitors. The names of all common medicines in these three groups will be found on pages 238, 240, and 242. The combination of nitroglycerine (in any form) and guanethidine can cause blood pressure to fall dangerously low. The same is true of the new group of medicines used in the treatment of angina, called the *calcium antagonists*. If you are taking one of these new medicines, you probably should not take guanethidine as well. If you have angina pectoris, you probably should not take guanethidine. *WARNING:* This medicine is very potent. The dosage must be adjusted carefully and slowly to make sure you do not experience too much lightheadedness or dizziness. If the dosage is too high, you will have a tendency to faint when you stand up. Be very careful not to become dehydrated or overheated when taking this medicine. Do not exercise vigorously without first taking a stress test. *Pregnancy:* Not proven to be safe. Do not use. *Breastfeeding:* Not known if it appears in breast milk. Do not use.

bethanidine (Banthid, Esbalid, Esbaloid, Esbatal, Tenathan) Comes in 10 mg, 25 mg, and 50 mg tablets. The intial dosage is 5 to 10 mg taken three times a day. The dosage should be increased no faster than about 25 mg per week. The usual dosage is 25 mg to 50 mg three times a day. For common side effects, important drug interaction, warning, pregnancy, and nursing, see guanethidine. Because bethanidine is shorter acting than guanethidine, it tends to have fewer side effects. For example, there is less of a tendency to be lightheaded on first getting out of bed. Diarrhea is also less of a problem, but it still occurs.

debrisoquine (Declinax) Comes in 10 mg and 20 mg tablets. The initial dosage is 10 mg twice a day. The dosage should be increased no more rapidly than about 10 mg per week. The usual dosage is 20 mg to 60 mg twice a day. For common side effects, important drug interactions, warning, pregnancy, and nursing, see guanethidine. Because debrisoquine is shorter acting than guanethidine, it tends to have fewer side effects. For example, there is less of a tendency to be lightheaded on first getting out of bed. Diarrhea is also less of a problem.

guandrel (Anorel, Hylorel) Comes in 5 mg and 10 mg tablets. The initial dosage is 10 mg three times a day. The dosage should not be increased more rapidly than about 25 mg per week. The usual dosage is 50 to 100 mg three times a day. For common side effects, important drug interactions, warning, pregnancy, and nursing, see guanethidine. Because guandrel is shorter acting than guanethidine, it tends to have fewer side effects. For example, there is less of a tendency to be lightheaded on first getting out of bed. Diarrhea is also less of a problem.

guanochlor (Vatensol) Comes in 10 mg and 40 mg tablets. The initial dosage is 5 to 10 mg a day. The dosage should not be increased more rapidly than about 10 mg per week. The usual dosage is 20 to 60 mg daily. For common side effects, important drug interactions, warning, pregnancy, and nursing, see guanethidine. It should be used with caution if you have any liver disease. Liver function tests should be performed before therapy is initiated and periodically thereafter.

guanoxan (Envacar) Comes in 10 mg and 40 mg tablets. The initial dosage is 5 to 10 mg per day. The dosage should be increased no more rapidly than about 10 mg per week. The usual dosage is 20 to 50 mg daily. For common side effects, important drug interactions, warning, pregnancy, and nursing, see guanethidine.

Methyldopa

methyldopa (Aldomet, Aldomet-M, Aldometil, Aldomine, Dopalin, Hyperpax, Medomet, Methoplain, Presinol, Sembrina) Comes in 125 mg, 250 mg, and 500 mg tablets. The initial dosage is 250 to 500 mg two to four times a day. The common side effects of dryness of the mouth and fatigue or drowsiness tend to go away after the medicine has been taken for a few weeks. Any other medicine which can produce sedation can accentuate the drowsiness caused by methyldopa. For example, alcohol, antihistamines, cold and sinus preparations, and tranquilizers may cause excessive sedation if taken with methyldopa. You need to keep this in mind, for example, if you drive a car. Methyldopa is very good to use in the presence of kidney disease. It tends to work best if given with a diuretic. Some men complain of inability to have an erection when taking this medicine. The problem goes away when the medicine is stopped. Nasal congestion and diarrhea are less frequent side effects. *Important drug interactions:* The blood pressure lowering effect of methyldopa may occasionally be prevented by one of tricyclic antidepressants listed on page 238. This is not a frequent occurrence but should be kept in mind since your blood pressure may go up if you are taking methyldopa and then add a tricyclic antidepressant. *WARNING:* Use cautiously if you have active liver disease such as hepatitis. Your liver function tests should be closely monitored. Methyldopa is known rarely to cause a severe anemia. You should have your blood checked for anemia about every six months. *Pregnancy:* Although methyldopa does cross the placenta, it may be safe. Use only if treatment of your high blood pressure outweighs the risk to the fetus. *Breastfeeding:* Appears in breast milk. Do not use.

Prazosin

prazosin (Hypovase, Minipres, Sinetens) Comes in 0.5 mg, 1 mg, 2 mg, and 5 mg capsules. Therapy should always be started at 0.5 mg to 1 mg taken once or twice a day, and the dosage should be slowly increased over a period of weeks. The usual dose is 5 mg to 10 mg twice a day. This is a very potent medication and you must see your physician frequently when you first start it. Lightheadedness or dizziness when you change position is the most common side effect, but that tends to be less of a problem after a few weeks of treatment. Headache, drowsiness, dry mouth, nasal congestion, and weakness are other side effects. It is generally most effective when taken with a diuretic. *Important drug interaction*: Use with caution if you take a nitroglycerine preparation to treat heart pain. The combination of prazosin plus nitroglycerine may cause the blood pressure to drop too low and lead to a feeling of lightheadedness and even to fainting. *WARNING*: This is a very potent medicine. Start therapy slowly, and be very cautious about your activity when you take the first dose. If lightheadedness or dizziness is pronounced, drink some liquid and stop the medicine until you can speak with your doctor. *Pregnancy*: Not proven safe. Do not use. *Breastfeeding*: Not proven safe. Do not use.

The Rauwolfia Compounds
There are numerous Rauwolfia compounds and many trade names for the same generic form. The reason for so many trade names is that the Rauwolfia compounds were among the first medicines effectively employed to treat high blood pressure. They have been around a long time, and many companies make them. All have about the same side effects, drug interactions, and warnings. The following table will help you to identify which one of the many Rauwolfia compounds you may be taking:

TRADE NAME OF RAUWOLFIA COMPOUNDS FOLLOWED BY
GENERIC (CHEMICAL) NAME

Agmaserp • reserpine

Agmawolfia • Rauwolfia serpentina

Alfolia • Rauwolfia serpentina

Alkarau • reserpine

Alserin • reserpine

Alseroxylon • Rauwolfia serpentina

Anquil • reserpine

Annaprel 500 • rescinnamine

Arcum R-S • reserpine

Austrowolf • Rauwolfia serpentina

Banasil • reserpine

Bonapene • reserpine

Broserpine • reserpine

Carrserp • reserpine

Cartric • rescinnamine

Cinatabs • rescinnamine

Cinnasil • rescinnamine

Crystoserpine • reserpine

Decaserpyl • methoserpidine

DeSerpa • reserpine

Ekans • Rauwolfia serpentina

Elserpine • reserpine

Eskaserp • reserpine

Geneserp • reserpine

Harmonyl • deserpidine

HBP • Rauwolfia serpentina

Hiserpia • reserpine

Hiwolfia • Rauwolfia serpentina

Hypercal • Rauwolfia serpentina

Hyperine • reserpine

Hyperloid • Rauwolfia serpentina

Hyper-Rauw • Rauwolfia serpentina

Hypersil • reserpine

Hypertane • Rauwolfia serpentina

Hypertensan • Rauwolfia serpentina

Hywolfia • Rauwolfia serpentina

Key-Serpine • reserpine

Kitine • reserpine

Koglucoid • Rauwolfia serpentina

Lemiserp • reserpine

Lesten • Rauwolfia serpentina

Loweserp • reserpine

Maso-Serpine • reserpine

Moderil • rescinnamine

Neoserp • reserpine

Protium • Rauwolfia serpentina

Rau • Rauwolfia serpentina

Raucap • reserpine

Raudixin • Rauwolfia serpentina

Raufonol • Rauwolfia serpentina

Rauja • Rauwolfia serpentina

Rauloydin • reserpine

Raumason • Rauwolfia serpentina

Rauneed • Rauwolfia serpentina

Raupena • Rauwolfia serpentina

Raurescine • rescinnamine

Raurine • reserpine

Rau-Sed • reserpine

Rauserfia • Rauwolfia serpentina

Rauserpa • Rauwolfia serpentina

Rausertina • Rauwolfia serpentina

Rausingle • reserpine

Rautabs • Rauwolfia serpentina

Rautensin • Rauwolfia serpentina

Rautina • Rauwolfia serpentina

Rautotal • Rauwolfia serpentina

Rauval • Rauwolfia serpentina

Rauwicon • Rauwolfia serpentina

Rauwidin • Rauwolfia serpentina

Rauwiloid • alseroxylone
        Rauwolfia fraction

Rauwistan • Rauwolfia serpentina

Rauwoldin • Rauwolfia serpentina

Ravadiscin • Rauwolfia serpentina

Rawfola • Rauwolfia serpentina

Rawiloid • Rauwolfia serpentina

Rawlina • Rauwolfia serpentina

Resedrex • reserpine

Reser-Ar • reserpine

Resercen • reserpine

Reserjen • reserpine

Reserpanca • reserpine

Reserpaneed • reserpine

Reserpatabs • reserpine

Reserpoid • reserpine

Resine • reserpine

Respital • reserpine

Restran • reserpine

Rolserp • reserpine

Roxinoid • reserpine

Ryser • reserpine

Sandril • reserpine

Sedaraupin • reserpine

Serenol • Rauwolfia serpentina

Serfia • Rauwolfia serpentina

Serfin • reserpine

Serfolia • Rauwolfia serpentina

Serolfia • reserpine

Serp • reserpine

Serpagan • Rauwolfia serpentina

Serpalan • reserpine

Serpaloid • reserpine

Serpanray • reserpine

Serpasil • reserpine

Serpasol • reserpine

Serpate • reserpine

Serpax • reserpine

Serpena • reserpine

Serpentina • Rauwolfia serpentina

Serpicon • reserpine

Serpiloid • reserpine

Serpine • reserpine

Sertabs • reserpine

Sertina • reserpine

Singoserp • syrosingopine

Tenserp • reserpine

Tensin • reserpine

Transerpine • reserpine

T-Rau • Rauwolfia serpentina

T-Serp • reserpine

Venibar • Rauwolfia serpentina

V-Serp • reserpine

Vio-Serpine • reserpine

Wolfin • Rauwolfia serpentina

Wolfina • reserpine

Zepine • reserpine

Reserpine is the one commonly used. It is the purest and most reliable of the Rauwolfia compounds. Reserpine comes in 0.1 mg, 0.25 mg, and 1 mg tablets. The initial and the usual dose is 0.25 mg once daily. It is long acting. The most common side effect is a sensation of nasal stuffiness which can be very annoying. You feel like you constantly have a head cold. If this occurs, stop the medicine and check with your doctor. It is also common to feel lethargic or drowsy when taking reserpine. If this side effect does not subside within a few weeks it may be best to ask your doctor to switch you to some other medication. Mental depression can be another side effect of reserpine. All of us suffer from mental depression at one time or another, but if your periods of depression seem unusually severe or more frequent or prolonged than usual, stop the medicine. Reserpine has also been reported to cause nightmares and unusual dreams in some individuals. There was once controversy as to whether or not it could increase the risk of developing breast cancer, but it has now been proven that reserpine does not do this. Reserpine may aggravate stomach ulcers. *Important drug interactions*: If one of the beta-blockers is given together with reserpine, the blood pressure lowering effect of the combination may be quite strong. Consequently, it may be necessary to reduce the dosage of reserpine if a beta-blocker such as propranolol is added to your treatment program. *WARNING*: If you have a strong tendency to be mentally depressed, do not use. If you become unusually depressed while taking it, stop and notify your doctor immediately. *Pregnancy*: Not proven safe. Do not use. *Breastfeeding*: Gets into breast milk. Do not use.

MEDICINES THAT PREVENT A BLOOD PRESSURE MACHINE FROM RECEIVING A SIGNAL

General Remarks: This group contains a number of quite similar medicines called the beta-blockers. Propranolol is the most widely used and best known of this group. One of the major actions of the beta-blockers is to cause the heart to beat more slowly and less forcefully. Consequently, when you take a beta-blocker, you should expect your pulse to slow down. Because beta-blockers slow down the rate of the heartbeat and also make the heart beat less forcefully, they reduce the work of the heart. For this reason, they are extensively employed in the treatment of angina pectoris. They must be used with great caution if there is any evidence of heart failure. Heart failure is a condition in which the heart does not beat as strongly as it should. Since the beta-blockers reduce the strength of the heart's contraction even further, they can induce or aggravate heart failure.

All beta-blockers have a definite tendency to aggravate existing asthma, emphysema, and severe bronchitis, and all can cause an old asthma condition to become active again. If you now have or have had a breathing disorder in the past, you should use a beta-blocker with great caution. If you now have asthma or have definite knowledge that you have had asthma in the past, you should not use a beta-blocker. A great deal of research has been done to try to eliminate the problem of possible breathing disorders. This has met with some success, and two of the beta-blockers (atenolol and metoprolol) which are now available definitely have less of a tendency to either induce asthma or aggravate one of the other disorders of breathing. Pindolol is also safer in this regard. However, no beta-blocker can be taken with complete safety if you now have or have had asthma.

Most of the beta-blockers are about equal in their ability to lower blood pressure, but they differ in the frequency and severity of their side effects. For example, if one beta-blocker causes bad dreams, hallucinations, or depression, it may be possible to take another beta-blocker and not experience any such side effect. Similarly, if one beta-blocker causes leg fatigue, it may be possible to substitute another which does not. By having more than one beta-blocker available, physicians now have some flexibility in finding the right one for you. The best choice, of course, is the beta-blocker that produces the fewest side effects and still allows effective control of your blood pressure. There is a great deal of individual variation in dosage of all the beta-blockers. Some individuals require (and tolerate) much larger doses than others. If your doctor has recommended a quantity of medicine considerably different from that listed below, do not be alarmed. As long as you are not experiencing untoward side effects, there is little reason for concern.

In the individual with only mild high blood pressure, a beta-blocker is often used without a diuretic. This is an especially common practice outside the United States, and it is a perfectly sound approach to the initial treatment of mild high blood pressure in the young. For older individuals and those who have more severe high blood pressure, both a diuretic and a beta-blocker may be required.

Propranolol was one of the first beta-blockers to be employed in the treatment of high blood pressure, and it is still the most widely used. It serves as the model against which all other beta-blockers are compared. For this reason, propranolol will be discussed first, and all the other beta-blockers will be compared with it.

The following table will help you to identify which one of the many beta-blockers you may be taking:

TRADE NAME OF BETA-BLOCKER FOLLOWED BY GENERIC (CHEM-ICAL) NAME

Anabet • nadolol

Aprobal • alprenolol

Aptin • alprenolol

Aptina • alprenolol

Aptine • alprenolol

Aptol-Duriles • alprenolol

Atenos • atenolol

Avlocardyl • propranolol

Beloc • metoprolol

Berkolol • propranolol

Betacard • alprenolol

Beta-Cardone • sotalol

Betaloc • metoprolol

Betaloc Duriles • metoprolol
(sustained-release)

Betaloc-SA • metoprolol
(sustained-release)

Betaptin • alprenolol

Betim • timolol

Blocadren • timolol

Blucadren • timolol

Cardinol • propranolol

Carvisken • pindolol (prindolol)

Coretal • oxprenolol

Corgard • nadolol

Deralin • propranolol

Doberol • propranolol

Dociton • propranolol

Gubernal • alprenolol

Herzul • propranolol

Inderal • propranolol

Inderalla • propranolol (sustained-release)

Kemi • propranolol

Lopresor • metoprolol

Lopressor Retard 200 • metoprolol
(sustained release)

Nedis • propranolol

Neptal • acebutolol

Noloten • propranolol

Obsidan • propranolol

Oposim • propranolol

Prent • acebutolol

Sectral • acebutolol

Selokeen • metoprolol

Seloken • metoprolol

Slow-Traskor • oxprenolol
(sustained-release)

Solgol • nadolol

Sotacor • sotalol

Sotalex • sotalol

Suminal • propranolol

Temserin • timolol

Tenormin • atenolol

Timocar • timolol

Timolate • timolol

Tracosal • oxprenolol

Trandate • labetalol

Trasacor • oxprenolol

Traskor • oxprenolol

Trasicor • oxprenolol

Viskeen • pindolol (prindolol)

Visken • pindolol (prindolol)

propranolol (Avlocardyl, Berkolol, Cardinul, Deralin, Doberol, Dociton, Herzul, Inderal, Inderal LA, Kemi, Nedis, Noloten, Obsidan,

Oposim, Suminal) Comes in 10 mg, 20 mg, 40 mg, 80 mg, and 160 mg tablets. The initial dosage is 10 mg to 20 mg two to four times a day. Usual dosage is 20 mg twice a day to 40 mg four times a day. Recent information suggests that propranolol may lower blood pressure just as effectively when taken only once or twice a day as it does when taken three or four times a day. (Inderal LA is 160 mg sustained-release). Consequently, it may be possible for you to simplify your treatment schedule, and you should discuss this with your doctor. Propranolol is often used in higher dosage in treating angina pectoris, and sometimes it is used in higher dosage to treat high blood pressure. The most common side effect is slowing of the pulse, which is to be expected. It can cause shortness of breath or wheezing in susceptible individuals. If breathing difficulty develops, stop the medicine and contact your physician right away. Propranolol can cause mental depression to develop and can make an existing mental depression worse. If you are depressed or have a strong tendency to depression, it may be best to try one of the other beta-blockers, because some may have less of a tendency to create or deepen depression. Propranolol sometimes causes bad dreams, depression, or hallucinations. You may find that your legs fatigue more rapidly when you take propranolol. Individuals often complain of cold hands or feet when they take this medicine. If you find that you do experience one or more of these side effects, ask your doctor to substitute one of the other beta-blockers. *Important drug interactions:* The beta-blockers and clonidine may counteract each other; each can make the other less effective in lowering blood pressure. Consequently, if you are taking one and then add the other, your blood pressure may go up; therefore it is important to have your blood pressure closely monitored to ensure that your blood pressure stays in good range. Use propranolol with care if you are also taking reserpine or any of the other Rauwolfia compounds, because when reserpine and propranolol are taken together, the blood pressure lowering effect of each may be enhanced and blood pressure may drop too low. *WARNING:* If your pulse rate consistently drops below 50 beats per minute, notify your physician. This may be a reason to lower the dosage. Do not take if you have emphysema or severe bronchitis, or if you have ever had asthma. If you have heart pain (angina pectoris) or if you have ever had a heart attack, *do not suddenly stop the medication.* Lower the dosage gradually over a period of about three weeks. Use carefully if you are being treated for sugar diabetes (diabetes mellitus) with either a pill (oral hypoglycemic agent) or insulin. Propranolol makes it more difficult for people who have diabetes to recognize when their sugar is getting too low. *Pregnancy:* It is now being used in pregnancy and may be safe. *Breastfeeding:* Gets into breast milk. Do not use.

acebutolol (Neptal, Prent, Sectral) Comes in 100 mg, 200 mg, 300 mg, and 400 mg tablets. Initial dosage is 100 mg twice a day. The dosage should be slowly increased over a period of weeks. Although it is commonly taken two or three times daily, once it is known that you tolerate the medicine well it can be taken as a single dose all in the morning. The full dosage is 400 mg. For common side effects, important drug interactions, warning, pregnancy, and nursing, see propranolol.

alprenolol (Aprobal, Aptin, Aptina, Aptine, Aptol-Duriles, Beta-card, Betaptin, Gubernal) Comes in 50 mg and 100 mg tablets. The initial dosage is 50 to 100 mg two times a day. The dosage should be slowly increased over a period of weeks. The usual dosage is 100 to 200 mg taken two times a day. For common side effects, important drug interactions, warning, pregnancy, and nursing, see propranolol.

atenolol (Atenos, Tenormin) Comes in 50 mg and 100 mg tablets. The initial dosage is 50 mg twice a day. The dosage should be slowly increased over a period of weeks. Once it is known that the medicine is well tolerated, the entire dosage can be taken once daily. The usual dosage is 75 to 150 mg taken all at once in the morning. For common side effects, important drug interactions, warning, pregnancy, and nursing, see propranolol. Atenolol is called one of the "selective" beta-blockers. This means that it definitely has less of a tendency than propranolol to induce a breathing disorder in susceptible individuals. However, it should not be used if you now have asthma or know that you had asthma in the past. ADDITIONAL WARNING: Atenolol is eliminated entirely by the kidneys. If kidney function is impaired, a toxic level can be built up in the body. Your doctor should assess your kidney function before you start atenolol, and kidney function should then be checked at regular intervals.

labetalol (Trandate) Comes in 100 mg, 200 mg, and 400 mg tablets. The initial dosage is 100 mg taken three times a day. The dosage should be gradually increased over a period of weeks. The usual dosage is 100 to 400 mg taken three times a day. For common side effects, important drug interactions, warning, pregnancy, and nursing, see propranolol. Labetalol has one property that the other beta-blockers lack. It has a tendency to directly dilate arteries in addition to its effect upon the heart and kidneys. Further experience is necessary to learn whether or not this is a helpful feature in lowering blood pressure in difficult cases and whether or not new side effects will surface because of this additional mechanism of action. It has one rather unusual side effect. It sometimes causes a crawling sensation in the scalp. This side effect soon disappears. Unlike the other beta-blockers, labetalol has been reported to occasionally interfere with sexual function in men, who can experience difficulty with erection and ejaculation.

metoprolol (Beloc, Betaloc, Lopresor, Lopressor, Selokeen, Seloken) Comes in 50 mg and 100 mg tablets. There is also a 200 mg slow-release form (Duriles or SA or Retard). The initial dosage is 50 mg twice a day. The dosage should be slowly increased over a period of weeks. The usual dosage is 100 mg taken twice a day, or 200 mg once daily of the slow-release form. For common side effects, important drug interactions, warning, pregnancy, and nursing, see propranolol. Metoprolol is called one of the "selective" beta-blockers. This means that it has definitely less of a tendency to induce or aggravate a breathing disorder than is true of propranolol. However, it should not be used if you now have asthma or know that you have had asthma in the past.

nadolol (Anabet, Corgard, Solgol) Comes in 40 mg, 80 mg, and 120 mg tablets. The initial dosage is 40 mg twice a day. The dosage should be gradually increased over a period of weeks. Once it has been determined that the medicine is well tolerated, the entire daily dosage can be taken all at once in the morning. The usual dosage is 160 to 240 mg taken once daily. For common side effects, important drug interactions, warning, pregnancy, and nursing, see propranolol. ADDITIONAL WARNING: Nadolol is entirely eliminated by the kidneys. If kidney function is impaired, a toxic level of the chemical can rapidly build up in the body. Your doctor should carefully assess your kidney function before you take nadolol, and your kidney function should be regularly checked while you are taking it.

oxprenolol, also spelled oxyprenolol (Coretal, Slow-Trasicor, Tracosal, Trasacor, Trasicor, Traskor) Comes in 20 mg, 40 mg, 80 mg, and 160 mg tablets. There is also a 160 mg slow-release form (Slow-Trasicor). The initial dosage is 20 mg to 40 mg taken twice a day. The dosage should be slowly increased over a period of weeks. The usual dosage is 80 mg to 160 mg taken twice a day. The slow-release form can be taken once a day. For common side effects, important drug interactions, warning, pregnancy and nursing, see propranolol.

pindolol, also spelled prindolol (Carvisken, Viskeen, Visken) Comes in 5 mg tablets. The initial dosage is 5 mg three times a day. The dosage should be increased about every two weeks as required. The usual dosage is 5 mg to 10 mg taken three times a day. For common side effects, important drug interactions, warning, pregnancy, and nursing, see propranolol. Pindolol has less of a tendency to induce or aggravate a breathing disorder than is true of propranolol.

sotalol (Beta-Cardone, Sotacor, Sotalex) Comes in 40 mg, 80 mg, 160 mg, and 320 mg tablets. The initial dosage is 80 mg taken twice a day or 160 mg taken once daily. The dosage should be gradually increased over a period of weeks. The usual dosage is 160 mg to 320 mg taken once or twice a day. For common side effects, important drug interactions, warning, pregnancy, and nursing see propranolol. ADDITIONAL WARNING: Sotalol is removed from the body by way of the kidneys. If kidney failure develops, a toxic level can accumulate. Your doctor should check your kidney function before you start sotalol and at regular intervals thereafter.

timolol (Betim, Blocadren, Blucadren, Temserin, Timocar, Timolate) Comes in 5 mg, 10 mg, and 15 mg tablets. The initial dosage is 5 mg taken two times a day. The dosage should be slowly increased over a period of weeks. The usual dosage is 10 mg to 15 mg taken two or three times a day. For common side effects, important drug interactions, warning, pregnancy, and nursing, see propranolol.

MEDICINES THAT TAKE OVER THE CONTROL OF A BLOOD PRESSURE MACHINE

There are four different medicines in this group: the diuretics, hydralazine (also spelled hydrallazine), minoxidil, and a new class of medicines called the calcium antagonists. The diuretics act by forcing the kidneys to eliminate salt and water; a diuretic is often taken alone to treat high blood pressure. Hydralazine, minoxidil, and the calcium antagonists widen the arteries. Hydralazine is usually combined with a diuretic; but hydralazine may be used without a diuretic when taken along with a beta-blocker. Minoxidil has a strong tendency to cause fluid retention and should always be taken with a diuretic. The calcium antagonists were first employed in the treatment of angina pectoris. This is still their primary usage, but in some countries physicians are now also using them to treat high blood pressure.

Diuretics

General Remarks: Along with a salt-restricted diet, the diuretics are the cornerstone of the treatment of high blood pressure. A diuretic is often the first medicine that you will receive after you have been instructed in weight reduction and a low salt diet. If your blood pressure is being treated with two or more medicines, one of them is likely to be a diuretic. Diuretics are among the safest of all the medicines used to treat high blood pressure. All diuretics have about the same action, but some are stronger and have a more prolonged effect on the body than others. Unless severe kidney disease is present, only one diuretic should be taken at a time. Combining two different diuretic medicines is seldom of any benefit in the treatment of high blood pressure except in certain cases to help retain potassium (this will be explained later in the chapter). You should always restrict your salt intake when taking a diuretic, because this makes the medicine more effective. If you eat salt while taking a diuretic, you can cause the medicine to become ineffective.

Many diuretics are strong enough and have a long enough duration of action to be taken only once a day. A strong diuretic is necessary if you have kidney disease, and the more severe the kidney disease, the stronger the diuretic that is needed.

There are two groups of diuretics. One group forces the kidneys to eliminate salt and water and is relatively strong. This group includes the thiazides, furosemide (also spelled frusemide), mefruside, ethacrynic acid, and bumetanide. The other group prevents the kidneys from retaining salt and water. This distinction is important, because the group that only prevents the kidneys from retaining salt and water is weak and, except in special cases, is not used to treat hypertension. This group is used to help the body retain potassium. It includes spironolactone, triamterene, and amiloride.

The weak group of diuretics is called the potassium-sparing agents. A medicine from the potassium-sparing group is frequently given along with one from the group that forces the kidney to eliminate salt and water. This is the only instance when two different diuretics are combined to treat high blood pressure. This prevents your body from losing potassium. The potassium-sparing agents are discussed further in Chapter 8.

No diuretic should be taken more than twice a day and *none should be given by injection unless you are hospitalized.*

The Thiazide Compounds. The thiazide diuretic compounds are the most commonly used diuretics in the treatment of hypertension. There are numerous thiazide diuretics and many trade names. All have about the same effect, but they differ in their strength and duration of action. The weakest thiazide diuretic that will do the job is the one that you should take, and one that can be taken just once a day is preferable to one that must be taken twice a day.

THE THIAZIDE COMPOUNDS (listed in approximate order of potency: weakest first, strongest last)

GENERIC (CHEMICAL) NAME	TABLET SIZES	USUAL DOSAGE
chlorothiazide (also spelled chlorthiazide)	250 mg, 500 mg	500 mg twice a day
hydrochlorothiazide (also spelled hydrochlorthiazide)	25 mg, 50 mg, 100 mg	50 mg twice a day
quinethazone	50 mg	50 mg twice a day
hydroflumethiazide	50 mg	50 mg once or twice a day
xipamide	20 mg	20 mg to 40 mg once or twice a day
benzthiazide	25 mg, 50 mg	50 mg to 100 mg once a day
chlorthalidone	25 mg, 50 mg, 100 mg	25 mg to 100 mg once a day
clopamide	20 mg	20 mg to 40 mg once a day
clorexolone	10 mg, 25 mg	10 mg to 25 mg once a day
bendroflumethiazide	2.5 mg, 5 mg, 10 mg	2.5 mg to 10 mg once a day
cyclothiazide	2 mg	2 mg once a day
butizide	5 mg	5 mg to 10 mg once a day
buthiazide	5 mg	5 mg to 10 mg once a day
bendrofluazide	2.5 mg, 5 mg	2.5 mg to 5 mg once a day
trichlormethiazide	2 mg, 4 mg	2 mg to 4 mg once a day
indapamide	2.5 mg	2.5 mg once a day
methylclothiazide	2.5 mg, 5 mg	2.5 mg to 5 mg once a day
polythiazide	1 mg, 2 mg, 4 mg	2 mg to 4 mg once a day
metolazone	2.5 mg, 5 mg, 10 mg	2.5 mg to 5 mg once a day
cyclopenthiazide	0.25 mg, 0.5 mg	0.25 mg to 0.50 mg once a day

The following table will help you to identify which one of the many forms of the thiazide type diuretics you may be taking:

TRADE NAME OF THIAZIDE DIURETIC FOLLOWED BY GENERIC (CHEMICAL) NAME

Acquarius • hydrochlorothiazide

Adurix • clopamide

Anhydron • cyclothiazide

Aprinox • bendrofluazide

Aquamox • quinethazone

Aquaphor • xipamide

Aquarius • hydroclorothiazide

Aquatag • benzthiazide

Aquatensin • methylclothiazide

Benzide • benzthiazide

Berkozide • bendrofluazide

Brinaldix • clopamide

Bristuric • bendrofluazide

Centyl • bendrofluazide

Chemhydrozide • hydrochlorothiazide

Chlotride • chlorothiazide

Clotride • chlorothiazide

Di-Ademil • hydroflumethiazide

Di-Chlortride • hydroclorothiazide

Dichlosuric • hydroclorothiazide

Diclotride • hydroclorothiazide

Diflumedil • hydroflumethiazide

Direma • hydrochlorothiazide

Diubram • chlorothiazide

Diucardin • hydroflumethiazide

Diucenin • hydroclorothiazide

Diuchlor-H • benzthiazide

Diulo • metolazone

Diuret • chlorothiazide

Diurexan • xipamide

Diuril • chlorothiazide

Diurilix • chlorothiazide

Diurone • chlorothiazide

Diutensin • methylclothiazide

Dixema • hydrochlorothiazide

Doburil • cyclothiazide

Drenusil • polythiazide

Duretic • methylclothiazide

Dureticyl • methylclothiazide

Edemex • benzthiazide

Enduron • methylclothiazide

Esidrex • hydrochlorothiazide

Esidrix • hydrochlorothiazide

Esmarin • trichlormethiazide

Eunephran • butizide

Exasalt • benzthiazide

Exna • benzthiazide

Flonatrel • clorexolone

Fluitran • trichlormethiazide

Flumen • chlorothiazide

Flutra • trichlormethiazide

Furane • benzthiazide

Hydol • hydroflumethiazide

Hydrazide • hydrochlorothiazide

Hydrenox • hydroflumethiazide

Hydrex • benzthiazide

Hydride • hydrochlorothiazide

Hydro-Acquil • hydrochlorothiazide

Hydrochlor 50 • hydrochlorothiazide

Hydrodiuretex • hydrochlorothiazide

Hydro-DIURIL • hydrochlorothiazide

Hydromox • quinethazone

Hydro-Saluret • hydrochlorothiazide

Hydro-SALURIC • hydrochlorothiazide

Hydro-Z-25 • hydrochlorothiazide

Hydro-Z-50 • hydrochlorothiazide

Hydrozide • hydrochlorothiazide

Hyeloril • hydrochlorothiazide

Hygroton • chlorthalidone

Igroton • chlorthalidone

Lemazide • benzthiazide

Leodrin • hydroflumethiazide

Lexxor • hydrochlorothiazide

Loqua • hydrochlorothiazide

Metahydrin • trichlormethiazide

Metenix 5 • metolazone

Mictrin • hydrochlorothiazide

Miuril • chlorothiazide

Miuzil • chlorothiazide

NaClex • benzthiazide

Naqua • trichlormethiazide

Naturetin • bendroflumethiazide

Naturilex • indapamide

Naturine • bendroflumethiazide

Navidrex • cyclopenthiazide

Navidrix • cyclopenthiazide

Nefrolan • clorexolone

Neo-Codema • hydrochlorothiazide

Neo-Flumen • hydrochlorothiazide

Neo-NaClex • bendrofluazide

Nephril • polythiazide

Novo-hydrazide • hydrochlorothiazide

Oretic • hydrochlorothiazide

Pluryl • bendroflumethiazide

Quenamox • quinethazone

Renese • polythiazide

Robezon • hydroflumethiazide

Rontyl • hydroflumethiazide

Salisan • chlorothiazide

Saltucin • buthiazide

Saluren • chlorothiazide

Salures • bendrofluazide

Saluric • chlorothiazide

Saluron • hydroflumethiazide

Sinesalin • bendroflumethiazide

Sodiuretic • bendroflumethiazide

Thiazidyl • methylclothiazide

Thiuretic • hydrochlorothiazide

Ufrix • buthiazide

Uridon • chlorthalidone

Valmiran • cyclothiazide

Yadalan • chlorothiazide

Zaroxolyn • metolazone

Zipix • xipamide

The side effects of all diuretics are related mainly to the strength of the medicine. The stronger the diuretic that you take, the more likely it is that you will experience a side effect. A sensation of lightheadedness or dizziness when you change posture is common. Use the rule: Sit Before You Stand. Stand Before You Walk. Occasionally these medicines will bring on an attack of gout in susceptible individuals. Your doctor may be able to tell if you have a tendency to gout by measuring your blood uric acid both before and after you take the medicine (see page 39). If gout does occur, it is not necessary to stop the medicine, but your doctor will want to add one of the anti-gout medicines to your treatment program. Occasionally these medicines will raise the blood sugar level. Your doctor should measure your blood sugar both before and after you start treatment (see page 38). If you have sugar diabetes (diabetes mellitus), the dosage of your diabetes medicine may have to be readjusted, a simple matter. Note as well that all diuretics can produce symptoms of potassium deficiency: which are excessive fatigue, muscle weakness, muscle cramps, and heart palpitations. If you develop one of these side effects, then you will need to take either a potassium supplement or a potassium-sparing agent (see Chapter 8). Men sometimes experience an inability to sustain an erection. This will correct when the medicine is stopped. Sometimes the thiazide diuretics induce a sensitivity to the sun. If this occurs, you are likely to develop a skin rash upon exposure to strong sunlight. You should keep this in mind if you break out in a rash, for example, while on vacation in a very sunny area. *Important drug interactions:* Diuretics must be used with care if you are being treated with lithium for manic depression. Lithium is made stronger when given with a diuretic. The dose of lithium will usually have to be reduced. The trade names of many lithium preparations are listed on page 242. *WARNING:* If you are also taking *any* heart medicine, such as digitalis, digoxin, or digitoxin, your doctor should follow your potassium level carefully. If you are taking a cortisone (steroid) medicine such as hydrocortisone or prednisone, your doctor should follow your potassium level carefully. (This refers to cortisone tablets or injections; you do not have to be as concerned if you are using a cortisone preparation on your skin.) Diuretics cause you to eliminate salt and water, and they have a tendency to dehydrate you. Any other condition that you develop that might also dehydrate you can cause lightheadedness, dizziness, or fainting. If you frequently experience any of these symptoms, stop the medication and check with your doctor. If you develop uncontrolled diarrhea or vomiting, stop the medicine and drink a salty broth such as bouillon or canned soups. If you sweat heavily because of excess heat or prolonged, heavy exercise, you may become dizzy or faint. Stop the medicine and drink some liquids. *Pregnancy:* Possibly hazardous to the fetus. Should be used *only* if the need for the treatment of high blood pressure outweighs the risk to the fetus, and should not be used as the only medicine to treat high blood pressure. *Breastfeeding:* Appears in breast milk. Do not use.

furosemide, also spelled frusemide (Arasemide, Dimazon, Dryptal, Frusetic, Frusid, Furix, Furoside, Impugan, Lasilix, Lasix, Seguril) Comes in 20 mg, 40 mg and 80 mg tablets. Usual dosage is 20 to 80 mg once or twice a day. Furosemide is a very potent diuretic and is used in the treatment of high blood pressure only when there is kidney disease. It is not used for the routine treatment of uncomplicated hypertension. The more kidney disease, the higher the dosage that may be required. For the common side effects, see the discussion of the thiazide diuretics. *Important drug interactions:* Lithium. See the discussion of the thiazide diuretics above. *WARNING:* Same as for the thiazide diuretics discussed above. *Pregnancy:* Known to cause fetal abnormalities in animals. Do not use. *Breastfeeding:* Appears in breast milk. Do not use.

mefruside (Baycaron) Comes in 25 mg tablets. Usual dosage is 25 mg to 50 mg given once or twice a day. It is essentially identical to furosemide; see furosemide for discussion.

ethacrynic acid (Crimaryl, Edecril, Edecrin, Hydromedin) Comes in 25 mg and 50 mg tablets. Usual dosage is 50 to 100 mg given once or twice a day. For a discussion of the common side effects of ethacrynic acid, see the discussion of thiazides above. Ethacrynic acid is sometimes used if you are allergic to furosemide. The reasons to use it are the same as those for furosemide. It is not routinely used in the treatment of uncomplicated high blood pressure. *Important drug interactions:* Lithium. See the discussion of the thiazides above. *WARNING:* Same as for the thiazide diuretics discussed above. *Pregnancy:* Not proven safe. Do not use. *Breastfeeding:* Gets into milk. Do not use.

bumetanide (Burina, Burinex, Butinat, Lunetoran, Primex) Comes in 1 mg and 5 mg tablets. Usual dosage is 1 mg taken once or twice a day. It is essentially identical to furosemide, but is about 100 times more potent. See furosemide for discussion. Bumetanide is of little value in the treatment of high blood pressure, because, although it is very potent, it is also very short acting.

Hydralazine (also spelled Hydrallazine) and Dihydrallazine

General Remarks: This medication works by forcing the arteries to dilate. It relaxes the muscles in the walls of the arteries. Hydralazine has been around for a long time and, when used properly, it is safe and effective. It should not be used alone, though. Generally, either a diuretic or one of the beta-blockers is used along with hydralazine. Whereas hydralazine makes the heart beat more rapidly, some of the medicines used to treat high blood pressure make the heart beat more slowly. For example, beta-blockers reserpine and guanethidine slow the heartbeat. By combining, for example, hydralazine and propranolol, the two opposing effects on the heartbeat are cancelled. Because hydralazine has a tendency to promote fluid retention, it is frequently used in combination with a diuretic.

hydralazine, also spelled hydrallazine (Aprelazine, Apresoline, Apressoline, Dralzine, Hydralyn, Hyperazine, Lopress, Rolazine) Comes in 10 mg, 25 mg, 50 mg, and 100 mg tablets. Usual dosage is 50 to 100 mg taken twice a day. The total daily dosage should not exceed 200 mg (see warning, below). Common side effects are headache, rapid heartbeat, and/or heart palpitations. If you suffer from migraine headaches, you are more likely to experience a headache. This usually goes away after you have taken the medicine for a week or two. The rapid heartbeat and/or a sensation of heart palpitations is generally prevented by always using hydralazine in combination with one of the other high blood pressure medicines that has a tendency to slow down the heartbeat, such as a beta-blocker. Hydralazine promotes fluid retention and usually a diuretic is required. *Important drug interactions:* None common. *WARNING:* Because hydralazine can speed up the heart rate, it may bring out angina pectoris if you have a tendency toward it. If heart pain or a sensation of palpitations occurs, stop the medicine until you can speak with your doctor. The dosage should not be greater than 200 mg per day. With high dosages, you may develop severe fatigue, severe joint pains, severe muscle aches, or a high fever. If any of these occurs, stop the medicine and notify your doctor immediately. *Pregnancy:* It is used in pregnancy and may be safe. *Breastfeeding:* Not known if it appears in breast milk. Do not use.

dihydrallazine, also spelled dihydralazine (Nepresol, Nepresoline, Nepressol, Pressaline) Comes in 25 mg tablets. It is essentially identical to hydralazine; see above for discussion.

minoxidil (Loniten)
Comes in 2.5 mg and 10 mg tablets. The initial dosage is 2.5 mg taken once a day. The dosage should be gradually increased about once per week. The usual dosage is 5 to 40 mg taken once daily. This medication is new and not all of its side effects are known. It should be used only to treat severe and advanced high blood pressure. Like hydralazine, it speeds up the heart rate. (See the discussion of hydralazine above). It should always be used with both a medicine that slows heart rate and a diuretic. One unusual side effect is a stimulation of the growth of hair on the face and extremities. The excess hair goes away within six months of stopping the medication. Women should be aware of this. *Important drug interactions:* Do not use with guanethidine. Blood pressure can drop

dangerously low. *WARNING:* Because it speeds up heart rate, it can make angina worse. See the discussion of hydralazine. The problems of possible severe fatigue, severe joint pain, severe muscle aches, or high fever which sometimes occur when hydralazine is taken have not yet been detected. It has been reported to occasionally produce a buildup of fluid around the heart. It is essential that you see your doctor frequently if you take minoxidil. If you suddenly start to feel short of breath, stop the medicine and call your doctor. If you suddenly start to gain weight, this probably indicates a fluid buildup. You should stop the medicine and call the doctor. *Pregnancy:* Not proven safe. Do not use. *Breastfeeding:* Not known if it gets into breast milk. Do not use.

The Calcium Antagonist Group
This is a new class of medicines, which were initially developed to aid in the treatment of angina pectoris. They act to directly widen blood vessels. Because they widen the blood vessels of the coronary circulation, they are of benefit to individuals who suffer with angina. This is presently their main usage, and it probably will remain so. However, in addition to widening the blood vessels of the heart, the calcium antagonists also dilate blood vessels in other areas of the body. Consequently, they are effective blood pressure lowering agents, and, in some countries, physicians are already employing them for this purpose.

Because they are so new, it is not possible to give you as much detailed information as has been provided for all the medicines previously discussed. They do constitute a significant contribution to the treatment of both heart disease and high blood pressure, and it is worthwhile for you to know about them. The following information will be of some help to you, but if you are taking one of these new medicines, you should ask your doctor to provide you with full information about side effects, important drug interactions, warning, etc., of the particular calcium antagonist that you are using.

TRADE NAME	GENERIC (CHEMICAL) NAME	USUAL DOSAGE RANGE
Pexid	perhexilene	100 mg to 400 mg twice a day
Bismethin, Elecor, Synadrin	prenylamine	60 mg three to five times a day
Cordilox, Ipoveratril, Isoptine	verapamil	40 mg to 120 mg three times a day
Adalat	nifedipine	10 mg to 20 mg four times a day

Some of the common side effects associated with the calcium antagonists include headache, heart palpitations, and lightheadedness upon changing posture. Important drug interactions: Use cautiously—if at all—with any other medicine that also dilates blood vessels, because the combination of the two may cause blood pressure to fall too low. For this reason, they should not be used with guanethidine or any of the related guanethidine compounds. If you have angina pectoris, be very careful about using nitroglycerin if you are taking a calcium antagonist. One of the major properties of all forms of nitroglycerin is that they dilate blood vessels. *WARNING:* Use with care if you have heart failure or have been treated for heart failure in the past. The calcium antagonists have a tendency to decrease the strength of heart muscle contraction and can make heart failure more pronounced. Use with great care if you are also using nitroglycerin, guanethidine or related compounds, or other medicines of the group that widen blood vessels. *Pregnancy:* Too little information. Do not use. *Breastfeeding:* Too little information. Do not use.

FIXED MEDICINE COMBINATIONS

All of the medicines described above also appear in various combinations. It is quite usual for someone taking medication for high blood pressure to take more than one medicine. If this is so, why not combine the medicines so that only one pill is taken? The only advantage to this is that it is quicker and easier to swallow one pill than several. The disadvantages tend to outweigh the advantages. First of all, a medicine combination is usually more expensive than the total cost of the separate medicines. Second, fixed medicine combinations do not allow your doctor to vary the dosage of each medicine separately to be sure that you have the most effective treatment with the least possible side effects. Fixed medicine combinations can be misleading. You should find out the names of your high blood pressure medicines. Are you taking any fixed medicine combinations? Did your doctor tell you that you were taking more than one medicine? You are entitled to know what goes into your body. Indeed, you should not take anything unless you know what it contains.

There are a large number of fixed medicine combinations. The following list is provided so that you can determine the composition of a fixed medicine should you be taking one. Once you know what is in your medicine, then you can use the information above to learn what you need to know about each of its components.

THIS BRAND NAME COMBINATION	CONTAINS THIS DIURETIC	PLUS THIS MEDICATION
Abicol	bendrofluazide (2.5 mg)	reserpine (0.15 mg)
Adelphane-Esidrix	hydrochlorothiazide (10 mg)	reserpine (0.1 mg)+ dihydrallazine (10 mg)
Adepresol	hydrochlorothiazide (10 mg)	reserpine (0.1 mg)+ dihydralazine (10 mg)
Aldochlor 150	chlorothiazide (150 mg)	methyldopa (250 mg)
Aldochlor 250	chlorothiazide (250 mg)	methyldopa (250 mg)
Aldoril 15	hydrochlorothiazide (15 mg)	methyldopa (250 mg)
Aldoril 25	hydrochlorothiazide (25 mg)	methyldopa (250 mg)
Aldoril D 30	hydrochlorothiazide (30 mg)	methyldopa (500 mg)
Aldoril D 50	hydrochlorothiazide (50 mg)	methyldopa (500 mg)
Aldotride (see Aldoril)		
Apresazide 25/25	hydrochlorothiazide (25 mg)	hydralazine (25 mg)
Apresazide 50/50	hydrochlorothiazide (50 mg)	hydralazine (50 mg)
Apresazide 100/50	hydrochlorothiazide (50 mg)	hydralazine (100 mg)
Apresoline-Esidrix	hydrochlorothiazide (15 mg)	hydralazine (25 mg)
Aquamox-R	quinethazone (50 mg)	reserpine (0.125 mg)
Bendigon	mefruside (15 mg)	reserpine (0.15 mg)+ inositolnicotinat* (150 mg)

THIS BRAND NAME COMBINATION	CONTAINS THIS DIURETIC	PLUS THIS MEDICATION
Bridina (see Brinerdine)		
Brinerdina (see Brinerdine)		
Brinerdine	clopamide (5 mg)	reserpine (0.1 mg)+ dihydroergocristine* (0.5 mg)
Brinerdine mite	clopamide (2.5 mg)	reserpine (0.05 mg)+ dihydroergocristine* (0.4 mg)
Briserine	clopamide (5 mg)	reserpine (0.1 mg)
Briserine mite	clopamide (2.5 mg)	reserpine (0.05 mg)
Caprinol	mefruside (10 mg)	reserpine (0.1 mg)+ methyldopa (125 mg)
Co-Betal	hydrochlorothiazide (12.5 mg)	metopocolol (100 mg)
Combipres 0.1	chlorthalidone (15 mg)	clonidine (0.1 mg)
Combipres 0.2	chlorthalidone (15 mg)	clonidine (0.2 mg)
Combipresan	chlorthalidone (15 mg)	clonidine (0.075 mg)
Darebon	chlorthalidone (50 mg)	reserpine (0.25 mg)
Darebon-mite	chlorthalidone (25 mg)	reserpine (0.125 mg)
Decaserpyl Plus	benzthiazide (20 mg)	methoserpidine (10 mg)
Demi-Regroton	chlorthalidone (25 mg)	reserpine (0.125 mg)
Dichlotride-S (see Hydropres)		

*This medicine has the ability to dilate blood vessels. It is an unusual combination.

THIS BRAND NAME COMBINATION	CONTAINS THIS DIURETIC	PLUS THIS MEDICATION
Diupres 250	chlorothiazide (250 mg)	reserpine (0.125 mg)
Diupres 500	chlorothiazide (500 mg)	reserpine (0.125 mg)
Diuromet (see Aldoril)		
Diutensen-R	methylchlothiazide (2.5 mg)	reserpine (0.125 mg)
Dopalin-H (see Aldoril) Dopamet (see Aldoril)		
Drenusil-R	polythiazide (1 mg)	reserpine (0.25 mg)
Durotan	xipamide (4 mg)	reserpine (0.10 mg)
Enduronyl	methylchlothiazide (5 mg)	deserpidine (0.25 mg)
Enduronyl Forte	methylchlothiazide (5 mg)	deserpidine (0.5 mg)
Esidri	hydrochlorothiazide (15 mg)	reserpine (0.1 mg)+ hydralazine (15 mg)
Esimil	hydrochlorothiazide (25 mg)	guanethidine (10 mg)
Exna-R	benzthiazide (50 mg)	reserpine (0.125 mg)
Hydromet	hydrochlorothiazide (15 mg)	methyldopa (250 mg)
Hydrometil (see Aldoril)		
Hydromox-R	quinethazone (50 mg)	reserpine (0.125 mg)
Hydropres 25	hydrochlorothiazide (25 mg)	reserpine (0.125 mg)
Hydropres 50	hydrochlorothiazide (50 mg)	reserpine (0.125 mg)
Hydro-Serp 25	hydrochlorothiazide (25 mg)	reserpine (0.125 mg)
Hydro-Serp 50	hydrochlorothiazide (50 mg)	reserpine (0.125 mg)

THIS BRAND NAME COMBINATION	CONTAINS THIS DIURETIC	PLUS THIS MEDICATION
Hydrotensin 25	hydrochlorothiazide (25 mg)	reserpine (0.125 mg)
Hydrotensin 50	hydrochlorothiazide (50 mg)	reserpine (0.125 mg)
Hydrotensin Plus	hydrochlorothiazide (50 mg)	reserpine (0.125 mg) + hydralazine (25 mg)
Hyser Plus	hydrochlorothiazide (15 mg)	reserpine (0.1 mg) + hydralazine (25 mg)
Inderide 40/25	hydrochlorothiazide (25 mg)	propranolol (40 mg)
Inderide 80/25	hydrochlorothiazide (25 mg)	propranolol (80 mg)
Ipotex	quinethazone (50 mg)	reserpine (0.1 mg)
Ismelin-Esidrex	hydrochlorothiazide (25 mg)	guanethidine (10 mg)
Ismelin-Navidrex	cyclopenthiazide (0.15 mg)	guanethidine (10 mg)
Metatensin 2 mg	trichlormethiazide (2 mg)	reserpine (0.1 mg)
Metatensin 4 mg	trichlormethiazide (4 mg)	reserpine (0.1 mg)
Naquival	trichlormethiazide (4 mg)	reserpine (0.1 mg)
Nortensin	furosemide (40 mg)	reserpine (0.4 mg)
Oreticyl 25	hydrochlorothiazide (25 mg)	deserpidine (0.125 mg)
Oreticyl 50	hydrochlorothiazide (50 mg)	deserpidine (0.125 mg)
Oreticyl Forte	hydrochlorothiazide (25 mg)	deserpidine (0.250 mg)
Prestim	bendrofluazide (2.5 mg)	timolol (10 mg)

THIS BRAND NAME COMBINATION	CONTAINS THIS DIURETIC	PLUS THIS MEDICATION
Prestyl	bendrofluazide (2.5 mg)	timolol (10 mg)
Rautrax Improved Sine K	hydroflumethiazide (50 mg)	Rauwolfia serpentina (50 mg)
Rautrax Improved 25 Sine K	hydroflumethiazide (25 mg)	Rauwolfia serpentina (50 mg)
Rautrax Modified	hydroflumethiazide (50 mg)	Rauwolfia serpentina (50 mg)
Rautrax Sine K	hydroflumethiazide (50 mg)	Rauwolfia serpentina (50 mg)
Rauzide	bendroflumethiazide (4 mg)	Rauwolfia serpentina (50 mg)
Regroton	chlorthalidone (50 mg)	reserpine (0.25 mg)
Renese R	polythiazide (2 mg)	reserpine (0.125 mg)
Repres (see Aldoril)		
Resaltex	hydrochlorothiazide (25 mg)	reserpine (0.125 mg)+ triamterene (50 mg)
Resertride (see Hydropres)		
Ropres	trichlormethiazide (4 mg)	reserpine (0.1 mg)
Sali-Presinol	mefruside (10 mg)	methyldopa (250 mg)
Salutensin	hydroflumethiazide (50 mg)	reserpine (0.125 mg)
Salutensin-Demi	hydroflumethiazide (25 mg)	reserpine (0.125 mg)
Sembrina-Saltucin	butizide (1 mg)	methyldopa (250 mg)
Serpasil-Esidrex 1	hydrochlorothiazide (25 mg)	reserpine (0.1 mg)
Serpasil-Esidrex 2	hydrochlorothiazide (50 mg)	reserpine (0.1 mg)
Slow-Trasitensin	chlorthalidone (20 mg)	oxprenolol slow-release (160 mg)

THIS BRAND NAME COMBINATION	CONTAINS THIS DIURETIC	PLUS THIS MEDICATION
Sotazide 160/25	hydrochlorothiazide (25 mg)	sotalol (160 mg)
Sotazide 320/50	hydrochlorothiazide (50 mg)	sotalol (320 mg)
Supres (see Aldoclor)		
Supres-150 (see Aldoril)		
Tenoretic	chlorthalidone (25 mg)	atenolol (100 mg)
Terbulan	furosemide (15 mg)	reserpine (0.1 mg)
Trasitensin	chlorthalidone (10 mg)	oxprenolol (80 mg)
Trasitensin Retard	chlorthalidone (20 mg)	oxprenolol slow-release (160 mg)
Trasidrex	cyclopenthiazide (0.25 mg)	oxprenolol slow-release (160 mg)
Unipres	hydrochlorothiazide (15 mg)	reserpine (0.1 mg) + hydralazine (25 mg)
Viskaldix	clopamide (5 mg)	pindolol (10 mg)

FIXED COMBINATIONS WITHOUT A DIURETIC

THIS BRAND NAME COMBINATION	CONTAINS THIS MEDICATION	PLUS THIS MEDICATION
Adelphane	reserpine (0.1 mg)	dihydrallazine (10 mg)
Adelphin	reserpine (0.1 mg)	dihydrallazine (10 mg)
Dralserp	reserpine (0.1 mg)	dihydrallazine (25 mg)
Serpasil-Apresoline 1	reserpine (0.1 mg)	hydrallazine (15 mg)
Serpasil-Apresoline 2	reserpine (0.2 mg)	hydrallazine (15 mg)
Trasipressol	oxprenolol (80 mg)	dihydrallazine (25 mg)

As you can see, there are numerous combination medicines available for the treatment of high blood pressure, and you can predict that as new medicines become available, even more combinations will appear. *Few of the combinations listed above are as effective as the proper dosage of each taken separately.* Many are of little value. To get the proper dosage of one of the medicines in the combination may result in your taking either much too much or much too little of the other medicine in the combination. The best use you can make of the tables is to learn you are taking a combination medicine so that you can request that your doctor switch you to individual medicines in the proper dosage range.

Some combinations of high blood pressure medicines have not been included in the above table. Many combinations end with the letter K. For example: Serpasil-Esidrex K or Burinex-K This means that the salt, potassium chloride, has also been added to the tablet.

In the next chapter you will learn that when it is truly necessary to replace potassium, a minimum of 20 mEq of potassium per day is required, and that it is common for an individual to require as much as 40 mEq to 80 mEq of potassium per day. It is not possible to obtain more than 10 mEq of potassium from a tablet. Consequently, you will have to take at least 3 tablets spread throughout the day to obtain even a minimal amount of potassium. It is important for you to know that sugar coated and enteric coated tablets are best avoided. If you do take a medicine that contains potassium in tablet form, it should be either a sustained-release or a slow-release formulation. Ideally, all the medicines required to treat high blood pressure should be capable of once a day administration, because this simplifies treatment and makes it less likely that you will forget a dose of your medicine. Only the liquid forms of potassium supplements are sufficiently concentrated to allow once a day administration. For this reason, and also because of their added safety, it is recommended that you initially use a liquid potassium supplement, and that you only change to a tablet form if you find the taste objectionable or experience an unpleasant gastrointestinal side effect. If you do take a medicine which contains added potassium, check with your doctor to make sure it is not one of the sugar-coated or enteric coated forms.

MEDICINES THAT ARE NOT RECOMMENDED

Certain blood pressure medicines have been shown to have dangerous or toxic side effects and have been removed from the market in some countries but not in others. Other medicines are still available but have been replaced by newer and more effective medicines which generally have fewer side effects and more reliably lower blood pressure. Still other medicines have added potassium, but no added K on the end of the trade name to let you know this. The following list will allow you to identify any which you may still be taking. If you find that you are taking any medication in the list, ask your doctor whether or not it might be preferable for you to be switched to one of the standard medicines discussed in this chapter.

Ansolysen	Mekamine	Rautrax N Modified
Arfonad	Mevasine	Repicin
Butiserpazide	Modenol	Revertina
Butiserpine	Pacepir	Ruhexatal
Butizide	Pentilium	Salupres
Caplaril	Pentoxylon	Selacryn
Cyclex	Perolysen	Seominal
Dalzic	Practolol	Sulfo-Serpine
Ecolid	Puroverine	Tenormal
Elfanex	Raupicin	Tensanyl
Eraldin	Rautractil	Thiaver
Eutonyl	Rautractyl	Ticrynafen
Eutron	Rautratil	Unitensin
Hypertane Compound	Rautrax	Unitensyl
Hypertane Forte	Rautrax D	Veriloid
Inversine	Rautrax Imp	Veriloid PB
Ipharon	Rautrax N	Versamine
Lasikal		

IS THERE A NEED FOR NEW BLOOD PRESSURE MEDICINES?

The medicines discussed above are generally safe, their side effects are generally well known, and they work. It is estimated that over 85 percent of all individuals who have high blood pressure can safely have it brought back to normal with simple medication. Unfortunately, the percentage of individuals who fully benefit from treatment is much less than this. It is tragic that of the many millions of individuals who have high blood pressure, a large proportion are not even aware that they suffer from this serious problem. Of those who have at one time or another been diagnosed and informed of their diagnosis, many are not actively being treated. It is estimated that less than one-half receive adequate therapy. Their blood pressures remain too high!

What is the reason for these unfortunate statistics? First of all individuals do not have their blood pressure checked with sufficient regularity. Next, when they do have it checked, they tend to neglect abnormal readings. Finally, physicians do not pay sufficient attention to abnormal blood pressure readings, and, when they do treat blood pressure, they often do not treat it properly. *These are the problems, and not inadequate medicines or too few medicines.*

As time goes on, new medicines will undoubtedly be developed to treat high blood pressure. This will be very meaningful to a small percentage of individuals who have very severe high blood pressure. It will *not* be very meaningful to the vast majority of those who suffer from high blood pressure. Newer and more potent medicines usually mean newer and more serious side effects. For those who really need such medicines, the benefits will outweigh the risks. For most individuals who have high blood pressure, the medicines already well known, those described in this chapter, will still be the medicines of choice.

If you have high blood pressure and it is not fully controlled, more than likely the solution to your problem is *not* a new medicine. You should not wait, hoping that a new and exciting miracle drug will come along before you take action. The solution is for you carefully to review your treatment program with your doctor. You now know how medications work, you know the logical way in which combinations of medicines are chosen, and you know about the medicines themselves. If your treatment program doesn't seem to fit the guidelines set down in this chapter, discuss it with your doctor. Sharing your concerns with your physician is the best way to guarantee that you will receive proper and effective care.

For the sake of thoroughness, two of the blood pressure medicines which are presently on the horizon will be briefly mentioned. The first of these, Captopril, is a member of a new group of medicines called "inhibitors of the angiotensin-converting enzyme," and it shows promise for those whose high blood pressure is not completely controlled by the conventional forms of therapy discussed in this chapter. Since it works by causing the dilation of blood vessels, it can be classified as belonging to the group of high blood pressure medicines that "take over control of a blood pressure machine." It works by preventing a natural body chemical, angiotensin II, from doing its job. Angiotensin II is a potent vessel constrictor. By preventing it from constricting blood vessels, Captopril, in effect, causes the vessels to dilate. As predicted, present studies reveal that there are significant side effects associated with the administration of Captopril. Since the medicine is new, it is likely that not all of its side effects have yet been identified. You should not anticipate that this new medicine or others like it will replace the old standbys.

The second type of medicine on the horizon involves the use of a group of chemicals called prostaglandins, which are naturally produced by the body. Since some of these are powerful blood vessel dilators, a great deal of research is now being done in an attempt to isolate prostaglandins that may be useful in the treatment of high blood pressure.

TYPICAL TREATMENT PROGRAMS

The Step Approach
You will remember that one of the guidelines in selecting high blood pressure medicines is to follow a stepwise program. There is

a logical sequence in which medicines should be added to bring down blood pressure and to keep it under control. Now that you are familiar with the unique three mechanisms by which a medicine can lower blood pressure, and now that you have some knowledge of each of the medicines that is available, you will need models of typical treatment programs to compare with your own. We will start with the simplest program and end with the most complex. Simple programs will control 85 percent of all high blood pressure cases. The more severe the blood pressure problem, the more complex the program.

Step 1. The simplest program is a salt-restricted diet plus weight reduction, if obesity is present.

Step 2. If the above does not completely control blood pressure, the next step is to add a diuretic. An example of a typical program is salt restriction plus weight reduction plus a diuretic.

Step 3. If the above does not completely control blood pressure, the next step is to add another medicine such as methyldopa, reserpine, clonidine, or a beta-blocker.

 An example of a typical program is (1) salt restriction plus weight reduction plus diuretic plus beta-blocker; or (2) salt restriction plus weight reduction plus diuretic plus reserpine.

Step 4. If the above does not completely control blood pressure, the next step is to add still another medicine, usually hydralazine or prazosin. Examples of typical programs are: (1) salt restriction plus weight reduction plus diuretic plus clonidine plus hydralazine; or (2) salt restriction plus weight reduction plus diuretic plus reserpine plus hydralazine.

Step 5. If blood pressure is still not controlled, then either substitute guanethidine for one of the medicines already in use *or* add guanethidine (or one of the medicines from the guanethidine group) to all of the others.

 Of course, there are other acceptable combinations. The choice of medicines will depend upon the initial severity of your high blood pressure, your ability to tolerate the various side effects, and your physician's own experience. Some physicians prefer some medicines over others. This is perfectly acceptable as long as all the medicines are used logically.

 Salt restriction is an essential part of *all* treatment programs. It is important that you learn to recognize the foods that are excessively salty so that you can eliminate them from your diet. The next chapter will discuss salt restriction and also the related topics of potassium-sparing agents, potassium replacement preparations, and salt substitutes.

DOES MEDICINE MEAN FOREVER?

Many individuals who have high blood pressure are reluctant to take *any* blood pressure medication, because they fear that once they start a medicine they will have to take it for the rest of their life. They fear they will become addicted to the medication and forfeit the possibility of trying to control blood pressure by salt restriction and weight loss alone at some future time. This is both false and dangerous thinking. Blood pressure medicines are *not* habit forming. If you start a blood pressure medicine, this does not mean that you must take it forever. It may be that after you have lost weight and maintained a low-salt diet (we will discuss the low-sodium diet in Chapter 8), you will be able to stop medication and have your blood pressure remain in normal range. If, when you do stop medication, your blood pressure rises, this does not mean that it is the fault of the medication. It means that your high blood pressure condition is sufficiently severe that dietary measures alone are not sufficient to keep it under control. It is far more dangerous to allow high blood pressure to go untreated than it is to take medication.

8

SALT, POTASSIUM, POTASSIUM-SPARING AGENTS, AND SALT SUBSTITUTES

Suppose the opening sentence of this book had been "If you don't eat salt, you probably won't develop high blood pressure, so put the salt shaker away now and stop eating salty foods." Would you have paid attention? Would you have taken this advice seriously? Probably not, even though telling you to reduce your salt intake is as important (if not more so) than any advice you have received so far.

Like all of us, you have learned to like your food a certain way and have learned to like certain foods. Changing a food habit is just that, changing a habit. And everyone knows how difficult changing a habit can be. Maybe you wonder if it isn't easier just to take a pill and go on enjoying your familiar lifestyle, especially since you are probably feeling fine.

The fact that high blood pressure is generally not uncomfortable is of course fortunate. Indeed, perhaps one-half of all the many millions of individuals who suffer this condition are not even aware that they have it. If you feel well, why should you bother to change the way you eat? Why take your medicine, for that matter? What is *less* fortunate is that by the time that high blood pressure does produce some discomfort, it is likely that the condition will also have caused some damage. Perhaps that damage will be minor and largely reversible through proper treatment. But why take that chance?

True, as proved in the last chapter, a "little pill" can probably do the job of controlling your blood pressure, but as the last chapter also shows, medicines are not without their problems. All medicines have the potential of producing annoying side effects, and these side effects may be more frequent and more pronounced when you eat salt. You now know enough about high blood pressure and its treatment to be convinced that "less is best." The following pages will make you understand the fundamental importance of salt restriction and prepare you to make the necessary changes in your own diet.

How Much Salt Do You Eat?

A level teaspoon of salt provides about 5 grams of salt, and one heaping teaspoon of salt provides about 8 grams. The average person eats between 6 and 18 grams of salt per day. Someone who salts food very heavily may eat even more salt than this daily. How much salt do you eat in an average day? One way to find out is as follows: Take a clean sheet of paper and lay it on the table. Pretend that it is a plate of food. Perhaps your favorite steak is on the plate, or a heap of delicious french fried potatoes. Pick up the salt shaker and shake salt on your pretend plate just the way you would if it contained food. Then carefully fold the paper down the middle and pour the salt into a teaspoon. How much of the spoon does it fill up?

Consider the number of times a day that you use the salt shaker. Now you have an idea of how much salt you *add* to your food. Of course, this doesn't include the amount of salt that may have already been added to the food by a food processing firm, and it doesn't consider the amount of salt that is in the food naturally.

Restricting the Sodium in Your Diet

When doctors and nutritionists speak of "salt" restriction, they really mean "sodium" restriction. It is the *sodium* content of our diet which plays an important role in the development of high blood pressure, and ordinary table salt is our major source of dietary sodium. What we commonly refer to as "salt" is the chemical *sodium chloride*, which is formed by the combination of sodium and chloride. (The chemical symbol of sodium is Na, and the chemical symbol of chloride is Cl. The combination of the two, NaCl, is table salt.) Sodium chloride is 40 percent sodium, so one level teaspoon of salt (5 grams) provides about 2 grams of sodium.

Salt restriction means sodium restriction. The average person eats between 6 and 18 grams of salt per day. This works out to 2.4 grams to 7.2 grams of sodium. A Moderate Salt-Restricted Diet should supply no more than *about 5 grams of salt or 2 grams of sodium per day.* A Strict Salt-Restricted Diet should provide no more than *about 1.3 grams of salt or 500 mg of sodium per day.* One gram (abbreviated gm) equals 1000 milligrams (abbreviated mg). As you will soon learn, it is quite easy to follow a moderate salt-restricted diet, but it is much more difficult to follow a strict salt-restricted diet. Fortunately, it is seldom necessary to more than "moderately" restrict your salt intake.

Where Does the Sodium in Our Diet Come From?

Sodium occurs naturally in all foods. It is lowest in fresh or unpreserved fruits and fruit juices (fresh, frozen, or canned), unprocessed grains, and vegetables (fresh or frozen but *not* canned). Eggs, unsalted meats, poultry, and all fish except shellfish are moderately low in sodium. Dairy products and shellfish have a rather high sodium content, and precooked and processed foods have the highest sodium content of all.

Although ordinary table salt is the major source of sodium in precooked and processed foods, it is not the only source of sodium. Many of the common foods that we eat have what is called *hidden sodium*. It is hidden because the foods do not taste at all salty. For example, baked goods contain either baking powder or baking soda, and these are major sources of sodium in our diet. A teaspoon of either baking soda or baking powder provides about 1 gram of sodium, which is about one-half of the sodium provided by a teaspoon of ordinary salt. A large number of prepared foods contain the flavoring agent *monosodium glutamate* (MSG, Accent), and a teaspoon of MSG provides about 700 mg of sodium.

In the United States it is estimated that about one-half of the food is processed in some fashion, and much of the world is rapidly adopting "the American style" of eating. Almost anything that is processed contains added salt. Some processed foods taste obviously salty. This is especially true of the many snack foods such as crackers and chips. More often than not, however, we are unaware that salt is present. Our taste buds have grown so accustomed to salt that we accept the flavor of foods as natural. Canned vegetables, prepared soups of all types, and precooked foods such as TV dinners and canned meals usually contain large amounts of salt. A cup of most prepared soups often provides as much as a gram of sodium, about the amount of sodium that is present in the ordinary can of vegetables.

Large amounts of sodium are found in cured meats. The sodium comes not only from the addition of ordinary salt but also from the addition of the chemicals sodium nitrate and sodium nitrite, which are added to prevent bacterial contamination and to give the pink color. Bacon, ham, luncheon meats, cold cuts, frankfurters, chipped beef, corned beef, pastrami, and smoked fish and meats are major sources of dietary sodium. One frankfurter contains 500 mg of sodium, and two slices of ordinary luncheon meat provide about 800 mg of sodium.

It is important to know that many of the common over-the-counter and prescription medicines are also significant sources of sodium. The common bowel conditioner, Metamusil, supplies about 250 mg of sodium per packet. Two Alka-Seltzer tablets supply nearly 1 gram of sodium. Many of the common antacids used to neutralize stomach acidity are high in sodium. For example, the common antacid Amphogel supplies about 25 mg of sodium per tablespoonful. Since it is common to use at least 8 to 12 tablespoons of an antacid each day, this can add up to as much as 200 to 300 milligrams of sodium per day. Basalgel Extra-Strength (22 mg of sodium per tablespoon), BiSoDol (420 mg of sodium per tablespoon), Titrilac (33 mg of sodium per tablespoon), Bromo-Seltzer (480 mg of sodium per teaspoon), Rolaids (53 mg of sodium per tablet), Creamalin (40 mg of sodium per tablet), Delcid (45 mg of sodium per tablespoon), Fizrin (673 mg of sodium per packet), antibiotics, and many other medicines your doctor may prescribe all can be important factors when you are trying to limit the amount of sodium in your diet.

The Moderate Salt-Restricted Diet
If you don't use the salt shaker *at all* and if you avoid many of the processed foods, you will still eat about one teaspoon of salt per day. This provides about 5 grams of salt or about 2 grams of sodium per day, which is the amount of salt allowed in a Moderate Salt-Restricted Diet, also called the No Salt Added Diet. It is very important that you change your diet at least this much. Although it will take some will power in the beginning, you will be surprised how rapidly you will become accustomed to it. Your taste buds will soon be quite sensitive to salt, and foods which once did not taste salty at all will soon take on a very salty flavor. Foods will take on new flavors, and you probably will find yourself enjoying the natural flavor of foods even more than you enjoyed the salty flavor. Salt masks flavors, and without salt your diet will have more variety.

The following is a list of the major foods and condiments which must be avoided in a Moderate Salt-Restricted Diet:

1. Salt. This means that any flavoring agent that contains salt must also be avoided. These include garlic salt, celery salt, onion salt, salt brine, sea salt, Season-all, Season-salt, Krazy salt, and Morton's Lite Salt. Sometimes the name is deceiving. You will have to read the labels to learn whether or not a flavoring agent contains salt. For example, lemon pepper actually contains a large amount of salt.

2. Many condiments and sauces. Most condiments and sauces contain between 300 and 400 mg of sodium per ounce.

These include ketchup, chili sauce, all bouillons, meat and vegetable extracts, relishes, and prepared mustards. Among the sauces which should be restricted are steak sauces, soy sauces, tabasco sauce, cocktail sauces, tartar sauce, Worcestershire sauce, and chili sauce. The commercial salad dressings should also be avoided.

3. Cured meats. These include bacon, ham, luncheon meats, cold cuts, smoked meats, corned beef, pastrami, and frankfurters. Some, but not all, kosher meats are cured by a process that adds a lot of salt to the meat.

4. Smoked and obviously salty fish. These include sardines, anchovies, herring, lox, and salted and dried cod.

5. Obviously salty snack foods. Anything that tastes salty or that has visible salt should be avoided. Many people are unaware that pickles, relishes, sauerkraut, and olives are highly salted foods.

6. Commercially prepared foods which have high amounts of "hidden" sodium. These include canned, frozen, and dried soups, TV dinners, canned and packaged gravies and sauces, shake and bake mixes, canned and packaged meals such as spaghetti, ravioli, stews, and pot pies.

7. Some foods served by the fast food restaurant chains which are very high in sodium.

If you follow the Moderate Salt-Restricted Diet, you may be able to bring a borderline blood pressure elevation down to normal. You should, of course, also lose weight if you are overweight. If this Moderate Salt-Restricted Diet doesn't completely control your blood pressure problem, your doctor will start you on medicine. If you follow this diet, you may require less medicine, and less medicine means fewer side effects.

The Strict Salt-Restricted Diet
If *many* members of your family are known to have or to have had high blood pressure, it is possible that the Moderate Salt-Restricted Diet will not be low enough in salt to prevent either you or your children from developing essential hypertension. If you wish to *prevent* high blood pressure from developing so that you can avoid treatment in the future, you and your family may be able to do so by following a Strict Salt-Restricted Diet. This will bring the total amount of salt that is eaten each day down to just a little over one gram of salt or 500 mg of sodium. To do this you must follow the Moderate Salt-Restricted Diet outlined above and also avoid the following foods:

1. Most dairy products. Dairy products contain a rather

high amount of sodium. An eight-ounce glass of milk contains about 125 mg of sodium, and when the milk is concentrated to make cheese, the sodium content rises significantly. Most natural cheeses contain about 200 mg of sodium per ounce (a slice of most packaged cheeses is 3/4 to 1 ounce). Processed, pasteurized cheeses have the most sodium of all, and an ounce of a processed American or Swiss cheese contains about 400 mg of sodium. This is over twice the sodium content of the same cheese not processed. Ice cream provides about 200 mg of sodium per serving, and margarine or butter provides about 100 mg of sodium per tablespoon. (It is possible to buy both unsalted butter and unsalted margarine.)

2. Canned vegetables. Canned vegetables usually contain five to ten times the amount of sodium that is found in the same quantity of either fresh or frozen vegetables.

3. Bakery products. Baked products are a major source of hidden sodium. A slice of the usual packaged bread provides about 125 mg of sodium. Five slices of bread exceed the entire day's sodium requirement. A tablespoon of margarine or butter plus two slices of bread will just about use up your sodium allowance for the day. A slice of fruit pie usually contains 300 to 400 mg of sodium, and this is about the amount of sodium contained in five good-sized cookies or a slice of cake.

This Strict Salt-Restricted Diet is obviously much more difficult to follow than the No Salt Added or Moderate Salt-Restricted Diet. You will have to carefully read the labels on all the packaged, canned, and baked foods that you buy to learn whether they contain any added salt, baking soda, baking powder, or sodium containing flavoring agents. In order to increase variety and flavor, you will probably want to purchase low-sodium or low-salt products, and this is an added expense.

Most individuals will probably not wish to follow a diet as limited as the Strict Salt-Restricted Diet. Fortunately, most will not find this necessary. If your blood pressure does not come down to normal after you have followed the Moderate Salt-Restricted Diet, it is quite likely that the addition of a simple medication will now allow effective blood pressure control with a minimum of side effects.

There may be some changes you will want to make in your eating habits even if you do not follow the Strict Salt-Restricted Diet. Perhaps you are someone who eats and drinks large amounts of dairy products. A quart of milk provides about 500 mg of sodium, and this is one-fourth of your daily allowance if you follow the Moderate Salt-Restricted Diet. Should you reduce the amount of milk that you drink? It is easy to eat a large amount of cheese, and cheese provides a great deal of sodium. It doesn't take many slices of pizza to add up to a lot of sodium! Because the processed, pasteurized cheeses have the highest sodium content of all, it will be best for you to avoid these and purchase the natural cheeses. Instead of canned vegetables, use frozen vegetables or fresh vegetables that are in season. It probably will be a good idea for you to cut down on the amount of pastry products that you eat.

If you have high blood pressure, you have a choice. You can moderately restrict your salt intake or you can strictly limit your salt intake. That choice is yours. You *do not* have a choice to continue eating salt and sodium-rich foods as freely as you now do. It is up to you to decide how much you wish to change your diet, but you must change your eating habits so that you at least follow a Moderate Salt-Restricted Diet.

Low-Sodium Foods So far you have been instructed to avoid many foods and beverages. Now some good news. Some foods are very low in sodium. Here is a list of foods and beverages that you do *not* have to avoid:

FOODS NATURALLY VERY LOW IN SALT	BEVERAGES NATURALLY VERY LOW IN SALT
vegetables, fresh or frozen	beer
fruits, fresh, canned or frozen	wine (table wines and dessert wines)
peanuts, unsalted	alcohol
pasta	soft drinks
rice	coffee
	tea
	fruit juices, canned or frozen but *not* tomato juice

Most herbs, spices, and extracts can be used freely. In place of salt, you can freely use one or more of the following flavoring agents to make your food taste more interesting.

EXTRACTS

almond	coconut	rum
anise	lemon	spearmint
banana	maple	strawberry
brandy	orange	vanilla
butter	peppermint	walnut
chocolate	pineapple	wintergreen
cinnamon	root beer	

HERBS AND SPICES

allspice
apple pie spice
arrowroot
basil
bay leaf
bitters
borage
burnett
caraway seed
cardamom
celery seed
chervil
chili powder
chives
cinnamon
cloves
coriander leaf
coriander seed
cumin
curry powder
dill seed
dill weed
fennel seed

fines herbes (parsley,
    tarragon, chives,
    chervil)
garlic (fresh, juice,
    powder)
ginger
honey
horseradish (salt free)
horseradish root
juniper
lemon juice
lemon peel
low sodium bouillon
mace
marjoram
mustard, dry
mustard seed
nutmeg
onion (fresh, juice,
    powder)
orange peel
oregano
paprika

parsley
pepper—(black, red,
    white)
pimiento peppers
poppy seeds
poultry seasoning (salt
    free)
pumpkin pie spice
purslane
rosemary
saffron
sage
savory
sesame seed
sorrel
sugar
sugar syrup
tarragon
thyme
turmeric
vinegar
wine vinegar (salt free)

Eating Out

Fast food restaurants are popular, but the foods that they serve tend to have rather high levels of sodium. Here is a list of the approximate sodium content of some of the more popular items served.

ITEM	AVERAGE SODIUM CONTENT
Hamburgers	
Burger King Whopper	990
Jack-In-The-Box Jumbo	1010
McDonald's Big Mac	960
Beef Sandwiches	
Arby's Roast Beef	870
Burger King Chopped	
Steak	965
Roy Rogers Roast Beef	610
Fish	
Arthur Treacher's	420

ITEM	AVERAGE SODIUM CONTENT
Burger King	970
Long John Silver	1335
McDonald's	710
Chicken	
Kentucky Fried 3-Piece Dinner	2285
Other Specialty Items	
Jack-In-The-Box Taco Meal	925
Pizza Hut Pizza Supreme	1280
Wendy's Chili	1190

On the basis of the above, the careful dieter would have to think twice before eating in fast food restaurants. Most regular restaurants do not add large quantities of salt to the food that they cook in their own kitchens, and now that you know which foods contain the most sodium, it should not be difficult for you to eat out and stay close to the limits set by the Moderate Salt-Restricted Diet. Here are some general guidelines:

BREAKFAST: Emphasize fruits, fruit juices, and cereal grains. (Although eggs are low in salt, the egg yolk is a rich source of cholesterol and it is recommended that you limit eggs to two per week.) Avoid cured meats such as bacon, ham, and sausage. Limit pastry products such as hot cakes, waffles, french toast, and pastries.

MIDDAY: Emphasize poultry, fish, and unsalted meats without gravy. Avoid luncheon meats, hot dogs, tuna fish, salted peanut butter, cheeses, and salted snack foods such as chips. Cooked and raw vegetables and fruits are excellent. Most soups will probably contain a lot of salt and should be avoided. Limit pastries and dairy desserts (sherbet is okay).

EVENING: Same as midday.

SNACK: Most of the processed snack foods are highly salted. Emphasize fruit, vegetables, unsalted nuts, and sandwiches made with unsalted meats and poultry. Choose only unsalted crackers and chips.

There are many surprises when it comes to the amount of sodium contained in food. Many foods which do not *taste* at all salty contain much more sodium than a very salty tasting bag of potato chips. You cannot just rely on your taste buds to guide you away from foods which are highly salted. You will have to read labels. As a rough guide, if the label states "salt added," you can assume it means "a lot of salt added." Here is a list of some common foods which all contain more salt than a bag of potato chips yet do not taste particularly salty.

ITEM	APPROXIMATE SODIUM CONTENT
Potato chips, 1-oz bag	*191 mg*
Jell-O Chocolate Flavor Instant Pudding, ½ cup	404 mg
White Bread, 2 slices	234 mg
Wish-Bone Italian Dressing, 1 tbsp.	315 mg
Corn Flakes, 1-oz	290 mg
Swanson Fried Chicken Dinner	1152 mg
Bacon, 3 slices	302 mg
Cottage cheese, low fat, ½ cup	430 mg
American pasteurized cheese, 1 oz	320 mg
Parmesan cheese, 1 oz	350 mg
Swiss cheese, pasteurized process, 1 oz.	388 mg
Kentucky Fried Chicken, snack box	728 mg
Canned spaghetti, 1 cup	935 mg
Canned vegetable soup, 1 cup	900 mg
Soy sauce, 1 tbsp.	1100 mg
Meat loaf TV Dinner	1200 mg
Waffle, 1	300 mg

POTASSIUM

Potassium is an important body chemical. The major symptoms of potassium deficiency are excessive fatigue, muscle weakness, and muscle cramps. The leg muscles are especially susceptible to weakness and cramps when a potassium deficiency exists, probably because they are the largest muscles in the body. The heart is also a large muscle, and it too is susceptible to potassium deficiency. In the presence of a potassium deficiency, the muscular contraction of the heart may become irregular. Instead of a steady, even beat, the heartbeat may become erratic. This causes palpitations or skips, and the pulse can be noted to be uneven. If there is no heart disease, the heart tolerates a modest deficiency of potassium quite well. However, if there is some underlying heart problem, the heart does not tolerate a drop in potassium as well.

Individuals who know they have a heart problem or potential heart problem must be careful to keep the level of potassium in the body at a near normal level, and this is especially important if any heart medicine is being used. For example, someone who is taking a digitalis preparation such as digoxin (Lanoxin) or digitoxin must have the potassium level watched closely. Since many individuals who have high blood pressure also have a heart problem, you can see how important it is to know about potassium.

A diuretic is one of the first agents that physicians prescribe when a medicine is required to control high blood pressure, and it is very often given along with *any other* medicine that is used to control high blood pressure. Diuretics directly attack the underlying cause of high blood pressure, and they are generally safer and have fewer side effects than many of the other medicines used to treat high blood pressure. Most diuretics can be taken upon getting up in the morning and their action on the kidneys will last until the next morning. This is a very desirable feature, since it is so difficult for most individuals to constantly remember to take their medications regularly. Diuretics are generally safe, convenient, and effective.

However, all diuretics cause the kidneys to eliminate some potassium. Although it is very desirable that diuretics force the kidneys to eliminate sodium—this is how it is believed that they work to control blood pressure—it is not so desirable that they also cause the loss of potassium, because many of the undesirable side effects that a diuretic can produce are related to potassium loss. Not only can a low potassium produce such undesirable side effects as excessive fatigue, muscle weakness, and muscle cramps, it can also aggravate certain important medical conditions. This is especially true of heart disease. A low potassium can make preexisting heart disease worse, and it can interfere with the effective functioning of the medicines which are used to treat heart disease.

If you have heart disease, and especially if you take a medication to treat heart disease, it is important to take corrective measures to make sure that your potassium levels remain in a near normal range. It may surprise you to learn that except in a few other special situations, most physicians now agree that it is *not* necessary to correct for the loss of potassium that diuretics produce. The reason for this is that except under certain special circumstances, diuretics cause only a relatively small loss of potassium, and this small potassium loss is ordinarily well tolerated by the body. It is not well tolerated if you have underlying heart disease, and it is not well tolerated if you take a heart medication. But unless you have a heart condition or take a heart medication, it is usually unnecessary for you to take *any* corrective action of any kind to compensate for the potassium loss which inevitably occurs when you take a diuretic.

No corrective action of any kind? Not even the traditional glass of orange juice or the ritual of a daily banana? There you are on the edge of your chair waiting to hear how important it is for you to eat or drink extra amounts of certain foods rich in potassium when you take your diuretic. Your doctor or your pharmacist may have made a special effort to advise you of the importance of such daily diet supplements. Giving you this advice is a well-established medical tradition, but it is a tradition which is without much scientific merit. If you do have a condition which makes it important that your potassium remains at a near normal level, you *cannot* do this by eating "potassium-rich foods" unless you are prepared to consume them in truly enormous quantities. For example, you must eat all the food that is part of your normal diet, and in addition you must drink the equivalent of about five 8-ounce glasses of fruit juice each day (which is more than a quart and provides about 550 *extra* calories per day), or you must eat the equivalent of about four bananas each day (an *extra* 525 calories). If you really do eat a sufficient quantity of potassium-rich foods daily to realistically maintain your blood potassium at a near normal level, you will rapidly become enormously fat. You could easily gain 30 or 40 pounds in a single year on such a regime!

Thus when it is truly important to correct for lost potassium, you cannot depend upon extra amounts of potassium-rich foods to accomplish this. If you take a diuretic and have a heart condition or take a heart medicine, dietary measures will not work. Similarly, you cannot depend upon dietary measures to replace lost potassium if you should develop symptoms of low potassium. In addition, certain special medical conditions and certain medicines accentuate potassium loss by the kidneys; if you have one of these conditions or take one of these medicines and *also* take a diuretic, you can lose extremely great quantities of potassium. The more common of the medical conditions which promote potassium loss are those which predispose you to retain excessive fluid. These include certain liver conditions and some forms of heart disease. Of the medicines which promote potassium loss, most are members of the steroid group and include hydrocortisone and prednisone. If you have one of the above medical conditions or if you take one of these medicines, it becomes important for you to take corrective action to protect yourself from developing an unusually low potassium. Eating potassium-rich foods will not provide you with this protection.

There is some minor controversy among doctors as to what constitutes an unusually low potassium level. The normal level of blood potassium should be 3.5 or greater. (The correct way to say this is, "3.5 milliequivalents of potassium per liter of blood." This is often abbreviated, "3.5 mEq/L." Don't worry. You will do just fine if you simply remember the number 3.5). Diuretics seldom cause the blood potassium to fall below 3.0 unless you are either unusually sensitive to the diuretic, have one of those medical conditions which predispose you to retain excessive amounts of fluid or take one of the medicines that accentuate potassium loss. Most doctors now agree that a potassium level of 3.0 or greater is perfectly safe and that a potassium level below 3.0 is potentially serious and should be corrected. *If your blood potassium falls below 3.0, you should take corrective action even if you feel entirely well, do not take heart medication, and do not have underlying heart disease.* Some doctors feel that this number should be a little lower, perhaps in the range of 2.7 or so, but 3.0 is a number which most physicians will agree is a reasonably safe limit for the blood potassium level.

How do you know if you are one of the individuals who are unusually sensitive to diuretics, whose blood potassium level may therefore fall below the safe level of 3.0? Unless you know that you have a condition which predisposes you to fluid retention or that you are taking one of the medicines that accentuate potassium loss, there is no way of predicting this in advance. For this reason, it is important for you to have your blood potassium level checked at regular intervals when you take a diuretic. How frequently should this be done? There is no absolute guideline, but once every six months is probably often enough.

Conditions That Require the Correction of Potassium Loss
Under most circumstances, it is unnecessary to take any corrective action to replace the potassium which is lost when you take a diuretic. This is so because ordinarily only a small loss of potassium occurs when you take a diuretic as part of the treatment of uncomplicated high blood pressure. Even this small loss should be guarded against if you also have heart disease or take a heart medication. Corrective measures should also be taken if you can predict in advance that you have one of the conditions which is known to be associated with an excessive loss of potassium. Of course, corrective measures should also be taken if you develop symptoms suggestive of low potassium, and this should be done even if your potassium is above 3.0. Finally, corrective measures should be taken if your potassium falls below 3.0, and the only way you can know this is to have your blood potassium checked at regular intervals—about every six months.

How Is a Low Potassium Corrected?
There are only two ways that you can realistically guard against a low potassium when you take a diuretic. One way is to prevent the kidneys from losing potassium in the first place. This is accomplished by taking what is called a *potassium-sparing agent*. Potassium-sparing agents act on the kidneys, forcing them to put back

into the bloodstream the potassium that would otherwise be eliminated in the urine. The other way to correct a potassium deficiency is to take in each day as much potassium as is being lost by the kidneys, and this is accomplished by taking what is called *potassium supplements*. A potassium supplement is a medication, not a food. Potassium supplements are a concentrated preparation of the chemical potassium, and they are taken like any other medication.

It is very difficult to eat a diet that is deficient in potassium. Almost all foods are rich in it. Meat, fish, poultry, seafood, eggs, fruits, and vegetables are all excellent sources. Ordinarily your regular diet will provide you with all the potassium you need to keep your blood potassium from falling below 3.0 but it is wise to confirm this with regular checkups. If the level of potassium drops below 3.0, remember that it is necessary to take medication, not food, to correct this.

POTASSIUM-SPARING AGENTS

You will remember from the previous chapter that there are two groups of diuretic medicines. One group forces the kidneys to eliminate salt and water, and these are relatively strong. They are the ones that are used to treat high blood pressure. There is another group of diuretics that are weak. These are not usually effective high blood pressure medicines when used alone. This second group works by preventing the kidneys from retaining salt and water, which is quite different from forcing them to eliminate salt and water. The medicines in this weak group have as their *major effect* the ability to help your kidneys retain potassium within the body. This group is said to be *potassium sparing*. Even though they do have a weak diuretic action, their major effect is to spare potassium. In certain cases, it is possible to treat high blood pressure with a potassium sparing agent alone.

It has been found very helpful to give a potassium-sparing agent along with a diuretic if you are unable to keep your body potassium at a satisfactory level (3.0 or above). There are three potassium-sparing agents that are available: spironolactone, triamterene, and amiloride. *Only one should be taken at a time. It is also extremely important for you to know that you should never take a potassium-sparing agent as well as a potassium supplement.* (Potassium supplements will be discussed later.) *It is also extremely important for you to know that you should not use a salt substitute when you take a potassium-sparing agent.*

Potassium-sparing agents prevent your body from losing potassium. If at the same time that you prevent your body from losing potassium, you also take in potassium in the form of either a potassium supplement or a salt substitute, your body potassium level can become too high. It is perhaps even more dangerous to have too high a potassium level in your body than it is to have too low a potassium level. Many salt substitutes are 90 percent potassium. All salt substitutes should be considered medication and not food. They will be discussed in more detail later.

General Remarks About Potassium-Sparing Agents and Potassium Supplements The three potassium-sparing agents are spironolactone, triamterene, and amiloride. They are often added to the diuretic agent used to treat high blood pressure when it is necessary to keep the potassium level in the body at a near normal level. You and your doctor have one of two choices:

You can take a potassium supplement, *or* you can take a potassium-sparing agent. Potassium supplements tend to have an unpleasant flavor, and this is the major reason why you might choose a potassium-sparing agent instead. Again, you must never take a potassium supplement and a potassium-sparing agent at the same time.

The major danger in taking either a potassium supplement or a potassium-sparing agent is the buildup of too high a concentration of potassium in your body. This is most likely to occur if you have any kidney damage. It is essential for your doctor to check your kidney function before either a potassium-sparing agent or a potassium supplement is given. This is done by checking your BUN and your creatinine (see page 38). If there is any evidence that you have kidney damage, these medicines should be used very cautiously. If there is evidence of *advanced* kidney damage, neither a potassium-sparing agent nor a potassium supplement should be used.

It is normal as you get older for the filtering action of the kidneys to decrease. This happens to *everyone*. Above about 60 years of age, potassium-sparing agents should be used with extreme caution. Diuretics usually do not cause the kidneys of older individuals to lose nearly as much potassium as younger individuals experience, so it is unlikely that most older individuals will need either type of medicine. If you are over 60 years of age, even if you have a heart condition or take a heart medication, neither a potassium-sparing agent nor a potassium supplement should be used until there is clear evidence that the diuretic is causing you to lose too much potassium.

POTASSIUM-SPARING AGENTS

spironolactone (Acelat, Aldace, Aldactone, Osiren, Osyrol, Urac-tone) Comes in 25 mg, 50 mg, and 100 mg tablets. The usual dosage is 100 mg daily, and can be taken as 25 mg four times a day, or 50 mg twice a day, or 100 mg once daily. The most common side effect is breast enlargement and breast tenderness in males. Some men complain of reduced sexual ability. This clears when the drug is stopped. Very occasionally, spironolactone interferes with the normal female menstrual cycle. This goes away when the medicine is stopped. *Important drug interactions:* Potassium supplements and salt substitutes should never be used if you are taking this medicine. See the general remarks about potassium-sparing agents and potassium supplements, above. *WARNING:* Do not use potassium supplements or salt substitutes. Toxic levels of potassium can build up in the body. Use with extreme caution if 60 or over. Do not use until your kidney function is first checked. Do not use if there is kidney failure. *Pregnancy:* Not proven safe. Do not use. *Breastfeeding:* May appear in the milk. Do not use.

triamterene (Diucelpin, Diurene, Dyrenium, Dytac, Jatropur, Na-trium, Noridyl, Teriam, Triamteril, Uretren) Comes in 50 mg and 100 mg capsules. The usual dosage is 100 mg given twice daily. The side effects, important drug interactions, warning, and use in pregnancy and breastfeeding are the same as for spironolactone. The major exception is that triamterene does not cause breast tenderness and breast enlargement in men, nor does it produce menstrual irregularities in women.

amiloride (Arumil, Colectril, Midamor, Modamide, Nirulid, Pendi-uren) Comes in 5 mg tablets. The usual dosage is 5 mg once or twice a day. Dosage should not exceed 20 mg daily. For common side effects, important drug interactions, warning, pregnancy, and nursing, see spironolactone. Unlike spironolactone, amiloride does not cause breast tenderness and breast enlargement in men, nor does it produce menstrual irregularities in women.

Fixed Medicine Combinations
Because potassium-sparing agents are often combined with diuretics to reduce the loss of potassium, a few fixed medicine combinations offer the advantage of taking one pill instead of two, but that is the only advantage. The fixed combination is usually more expensive than the total cost of the two separate medicines, and your doctor does not have the option to alter the dosage of one and not the other. For your information, the fixed combinations of a potassium-sparing agent and a diuretic which are available include:

THIS BRAND NAME COMBINATION	CONTAINS THIS POTASSIUM-SPARING AGENT	PLUS THIS DIURETIC
Aldactazida	spironolactone (25 mg)	hydrochlorothiazide (25 mg)
Aldactazide	spironolactone (25 mg)	hydrochlorthiazide (25 mg)
Aldactide 25	spironolactone (25 mg)	hydroflumethiazide (25 mg)
Aldactide 50	spironolactone (50 mg)	hydroflumethiazide (50 mg)
Aldazide	spironolactone (25 mg)	thiabutazide (2.5 mg)
Dyazide	triamterene (50 mg)	hydrochlorthiazide (25 mg)
Dytide	triamterene (50 mg)	benzthiazide (25 mg)
Moduretic	amiloride (5 mg)	hydrochlorthiazide (50 mg)
Resaltex	triamterene (50 mg)	reserpine (0.125 mg) plus hydrochlorthiazide (25 mg)

POTASSIUM SUPPLEMENTS

Potassium supplements are medicines which are used to replace potassium when an individual who takes a diuretic cannot maintain a satisfactory level of potassium in the body or has one of the conditions which makes it important to keep the body's potassium in near normal range. Potassium supplements should never be used along with a potassium-sparing agent. The choice of whether to take a potassium supplement or a potassium-sparing agent is generally a matter of personal preference. Remember that salt substitutes contain potassium and should be used with great care (if at all) when you are taking any form of potassium supplement.

General Remarks About Potassium Supplements There are a variety of potassium supplements on the market. The oldest and most widely prescribed are those that either are already in liquid form or which are *fully dissolved* in liquid before taking. The liquid forms of potassium are generally safe, and they contain potassium in sufficient concentration to be taken just once or twice a day. Potassium has a bitter taste, and the pharmaceutical companies have made a real effort to discover flavoring agents to add to the liquid forms to make them palatable. There are numerous brands of liquid potassium available, and if you find the taste of one brand to be objectionable, you might be able to find another that you can tolerate. All liquid forms of potassium have the potential of causing gastrointestinal side effects such as nausea, a burning sensation in the stomach, or indigestion. These gastrointestinal side effects are unrelated to the flavor of the liquid potassium supplements; they are a consequence of dosage. Concentrated potassium is irritating to the tissues, and the more concentrated the liquid potassium, the more likely it is that it will produce a disagreeable side effect. No form of liquid potassium supplement can be taken undiluted. Those that are already in a liquid form must be further diluted with liquid before taking, and those that are in tablet or powder form must first be diluted before taking. It may be possible to overcome the gastrointestinal distress produced by a liquid potassium preparation by further diluting before drinking. You can use water, fruit juice, or almost any other liquid for this purpose. The flavor of the liquid that you choose to dilute the potassium supplement may help to improve its flavor.

Potassium tablets were developed to overcome the problems of taste and gastrointestinal upset associated with the liquid potassium supplements. There are four types of potassium tablets: sugar coated, enteric coated, slow-release, and sustained-release. Sugar coated tablets simply have a covering of compressed sugar to improve taste. and they usually dissolve in the stomach. Because they dissolve in the stomach, they can produce the same gastrointestinal side effects as the liquids. Should they *not* dissolve in the stomach, they can produce ulceration of the tissue. This is a potentially serious side effect, and it will be discussed shortly. Enteric coated tablets have an especially designed coating which allows them to pass through the stomach intact and dissolve in the small intestine. This property avoids the problem of nausea or an upset stomach, but has been shown to be associated with a significant incidence of tissue ulceration. The slow-release and sustained-release tablets were developed to overcome this very serious side effect. They, too, are designed to pass through the stomach unchanged, but their potassium is released into the intestine more gradually and more reliably than is true of either the enteric coated or the sugar coated tablets. The potential problem of intestinal ulceration still exists with the slow-release and the sustained-release tablets, but it is a very infrequent event.

In concentrated form, potassium is very irritating to tissues. If the passage of any form of potassium tablet is delayed after it is swallowed, the danger exists that all of its potassium will be released at one location. This can so irritate the tissues that an ulcer develops. If the ulcer is sufficiently deep, perforation of the intestine is possible. Even if the ulcer does not perforate, its healing presents a problem, because healing is often associated with the formation of scar tissue. If scar tissue develops at the site of the former ulcer, a portion of the intestine can become narrowed or entirely blocked.

Ulceration of tissue is most likely to occur with the enteric and sugar coated tablets, and most physicians agree that they are best avoided. The slow-release and the sustained-release tablets are so formulated that ulceration seldom occurs. Because this potentially serious side effect is not completely eliminated, some physicians are reluctant to recommend even the slow-release and sustained-release tablets. However, most physicians believe them to be safe as long as you do not have a condition which could cause a delay in the passage of the tablet through the esophagus, stomach, or intestine.

There is one problem that is associated with the enteric coated tablets that is avoided by all other potassium supplements. It is possible for an enteric coated tablet to pass through the intestine without dissolving at all. This does the intestine no harm, but it does mean that less potassium is taken into the body than anticipated. This creates a false sense of security and can lead to an unsuspected potassium deficiency.

Since the liquid forms of potassium are equally as effective as the tablet forms and are associated with less serious side effects, it is suggested that you start with one of the liquids should you choose a potassium supplement over a potassium-sparing agent. If one brand of liquid potassium has an unpleasant taste, try another. If you experience nausea or an upset stomach, try diluting the liquid potassium with a greater volume of liquid. If you still find you cannot tolerate a liquid potassium, then you have the option of using either a slow-release or sustained-release tablet or a potassium-sparing agent. Which to choose? If your doctor can assure you that you do not have a condition which might cause a tablet to become slowed during its passage through your esophagus, stomach, or small intestine, the slow-release and sustained-release tablets should be as safe as the potassium-sparing agents. The tablets only contain between 6.67 mEq to 10.0 mEq of potassium per tablet. Some individuals require as much as 60 mEq to 80 mEq of potassium per day when they take a diuretic and have to take anywhere from 6 to 12 tablets. If you require a fairly large quantity of potassium each day, you may prefer a potassium-sparing agent to avoid taking so many pills.

Most potassium supplements come as potassium chloride. Occasionally, other salts of potassium are used, such as potassium acetate, potassium carbonate, potassium citrate, or potassium gluconate. The advantage of these other salts over the potassium chloride salt is their better taste. The disadvantage is that they do not do as effective a job of replacing the body's potassium. When a diuretic causes the kidney to lose potassium, it also causes the kidney to lose chloride, and it is often difficult to fully correct a low potassium level unless the chloride level is also corrected. Consequently, the chloride forms are recommended. It is better to sacrifice somewhat on taste for the extra assurance that your metabolism remains in satisfactory balance.

Potassium Supplements in Liquid Form

• Liquid potassium chloride (Cena-K, Kaochlor 10%, Kaochlor SF, Kaon-Cl 20%, Kay-Cee-L, Kay Ciel Elixir, Klor 10%, K-Lor 10%, Klor-Con 20%, Kloride Elixir, Klorvess 10%, Kolyum liquid, PfiKlor 10%, Rum K).

    • Powder and tablet forms of potassium chloride, to be fully dissolved in liquid before taking (Kaochlor-Eff, Kato Powder, Kay Ciel Powder Solodose, Keff, Klor-Con, K-Lor, Klorvess, K-Lyte/CL, PfiKlor Powder).

    • Liquid potassium other than the chloride salt (Kajos, Kalinate, Kaon Elixir, Katorin, K-Lyte, Kolyum Liquid, Potassium Oligosol, Potassium Rougier, Potassium Tiplex, Twin-K).

    • Powder and tablet forms of potassium other than the chloride, to be completely dissolved in liquid before taking (Kloref, Kloref-S, K-Lyte, K-Lyte/DS, Kolyum Powder, K-Sandoz, PfiKlor-F Effervescent Tablets, Sando-K).

    The liquids provide 20 mEq of potassium per tablespoon, except Kaon-Cl 20%, which provides 40 mEq of potassium per tablespoon. The fully dissolvable powders and tablets usually provide either 20 mEq or 25 mEq of potassium per dose. K-Lyte/DS and K-Lyte/CL each provides 50 mg of potassium per dose. The usual dose of a potassium supplement is 20 mEq to 40 mEq per day, but it is not unusual for an individual who develops a significant potassium deficiency or who is very sensitive to diuretics to require 60 mEq to 80 mEq per day. The common side effect is bitter taste of the medicine. Abdominal discomfort, nausea, vomiting, and diarrhea are less common side effects. *Important drug interactions:* Do not use potassium-sparing agents (triamterene, amiloride, and spironolactone) or salt substitutes while taking a potassium supplement. *WARNING:* See the warning for potassium-sparing agents. *Pregnancy:* Safe to use. *Breastfeeding:* Safe to use.

Potassium Supplements, Tablet Form

• Potassium chloride tablets that do not dissolve before taking (Kalium Durules, Kaon-Cl, K-Contin, Leo K, Slow-K, Span-K).

    • Potassium tablets other than the chloride (Kaon).

    The tablets provide between 6.67 mEq potassium (Kaon-Cl) to 10 mEq potassium (Kalium Durules) per tablet. Usual dosage is four to six tablets per day. The side effect is intestinal ulceration. *Important drug interactions:* See the discussion of liquid potassium above. *WARNING:* Can cause intestinal ulcers. Also see *WARNING* for potassium sparing agents, page 112. *Pregnancy:* Safe for fetus. *Breastfeeding:* Safe for baby.

SALT SUBSTITUTES

Salt substitutes are not prescription items. They can be purchased in food stores and pharmacies. They were developed to give individuals who need to follow a salt-restricted diet something to sprinkle on food to give it somewhat of a salty flavor. This is a good idea in principle, but in fact these seemingly innocuous "foods" are potentially dangerous. Most salt substitutes are about 90 percent potassium chloride. *One teaspoon of a salt substitute can contain up to 135 mEq of potassium chloride.* You just learned that the usual dosage of a potassium supplement is 20 to 40 mEq per day. One teaspoon of a salt substitute can provide up to *three times* the daily recommended dose of a legitimate prescription-controlled potassium supplement. The salt substitutes are particularly hazardous to children, older adults, and anyone who has kidney damage. Salt substitutes must be used with care. They must not be used if you are also taking either a potassium-sparing agent or a potassium supplement. They don't taste that much like real salt anyway. Instead of getting used to the taste of a salt substitute, consider getting used to the taste of food without added salt!

The following salt substitutes are 90 percent potassium chloride: Co-Salt, Feather-weight K, Neocurtasal, Nu-Salt, and Selora. Morton's Lite Salt is 50 percent potassium chloride and 50 percent sodium chloride. Ruthmol is 50 percent potassium chloride and 50 percent inert base.

9

THE TREATMENT OF HIGH BLOOD PRESSURE WITH SURGERY

Occasionally an adult will have a form of high blood pressure which can be permanently cured by an operation. Although such a condition is uncommon, it is worth identifying, because the underlying diseases which cause surgically correctable hypertension are all quite serious and medications often are not completely effective in controlling them. A knowledgeable physician who performs a careful medical interview, a thorough physical examination, and the basic set of laboratory tests is unlikely to overlook the clues which will be present if you do have one of the five diseases that cause surgically correctable high blood pressure. If you have been properly evaluated and your doctor has told you that you have "essential" or "primary" hypertension, don't worry. It is extremely unlikely that you have one of these diseases. You still might like to read this chapter because the indications for performing an IVP (intravenous pyelogram) and an arteriogram—procedures which you or a member of your family might undergo for other reasons—will also be discussed along with the potential complications of these important diagnostic tests.

What clues might your doctor discover during the routine medical evaluation of high blood pressure to suggest that you may be one of the unusual individuals who has a narrowed artery to the kidney, or hyperaldosteronism, or Cushing's disease, or pheochromocytoma, or coarctation of the aorta? When should you have further diagnostic tests such as an X-ray of the kidneys (IVP), or an X-ray of the arteries (arteriogram), or a 24-hour urine collection for chemical analysis? Is hospitalization necessary? How are the tests performed? Are they uncomfortable? Are there potential complications? Should your doctor obtain the assistance of an endocrinologist?

NARROWING OF THE MAJOR ARTERY TO A KIDNEY (RENAL ARTERY STENOSIS)

In Chapter 6 you learned that a kidney may cause high blood pressure when it suffers a reduction in its blood supply. The kidney is not able to understand that the reduction in its blood flow is only a local problem. Even though the remainder of the circulatory system is quite normal and only the blood supply to the kidney is impaired, this blood pressure regulating machine believes that there is a need to raise the blood pressure, and it inappropriately gets its machinery going to accomplish this task. The kidney senses its reduction in blood flow to be an overwhelming threat to the entire body. It ignores the message from the nervous system which tells it that all is fine elsewhere, and because it is a very effective blood pressure regulatory machine, its hard work soon results in a sustained and serious high blood pressure condition.

RENAL ARTERY STENOSIS VS SMALL VESSEL DISEASE

There are two ways that the kidney can suffer a reduction in its blood supply: the large artery which brings blood into the kidney can become narrowed, or the small blood vessels within the kidney can develop numerous tiny obstructions. Of course, both processes can occur simultaneously. No matter how the problem arises, the end result—high blood pressure—is the same. However, the treatment of the two conditions is different. High blood pressure due to small vessel disease is always treated with medicines, but high blood pressure produced by a narrowed renal artery (renal artery stenosis) is often best treated by surgery. Because the treatment of these two conditions is often different, it becomes important for your doctor to be able to distinguish one from the other.

Small Vessel Disease
Probably the most common cause of small vessel disease of the kidneys is high blood pressure itself. Like all arteries, the arteries within the kidneys are susceptible to the process called *atherosclerosis*. Deposits of cholesterol and fat build up in the walls of the arteries to cause narrowing and, at times, complete obstruction. (The causes and prevention of atherosclerosis are discussed at length in Chapter 16.) It is not surprising that high blood pressure is a major cause of atherosclerosis, because the high pressure damages the walls of the arteries and makes them more susceptible to the deposition of fat and cholesterol. This process usually occurs

slowly over a period of years, but the more severe the high blood pressure condition, the more rapidly it will occur. Eventually, the blood supply to thc kidneys becomes sufficiently reduced that the kidneys begin inappropriately to raise the blood pressure.

When the kidney raises the blood pressure, this does not mean that more blood will come to the kidneys and correct their blood supply problem. In fact, just the opposite can occur. When the problem is due to damage to small blood vessels within the kidneys, all that happens when the blood pressure goes up is that these small vessels become even further damaged. This further damage to the blood vessels results in an even further rise in blood pressure. A vicious cycle can develop: more damage to blood vessels causes more rise in blood pressure causes more damage to blood vessels, and so on.

In this situation it is absolutely essential that medication to treat high blood pressure be started as early as possible. When high blood pressure is caused by *small vessel disease*, treatment with medication does more than just control the blood pressure. It also protects the kidneys from further damage to the small blood vessels. If the cycle of blood vessel damage leading to high blood pressure leading to more blood vessel damage is not arrested, eventually the blood supply to the kidneys will become inadequate, and kidney failure will result.

Untreated high blood pressure is a leading cause of kidney failure. Now you know why. As the blood vessels within the kidney become progressively damaged by the high blood pressure condition, eventually the ability of the kidneys to filter and purify the blood will be impaired. As the kidneys progressively lose their blood supply, they also progressively lose their ability to function. There is a progressive loss of kidney tissue. The kidneys become smaller and smaller and less capable of doing their job.

Fortunately, treatment of high blood pressure with medication is extremely effective in preventing this progressive damage to the kidneys. High blood pressure medicine, in controlling the blood pressure, does more than just bring blood pressure down to normal and keep it there. It breaks the vicious cycle of high blood pressure leading to atherosclerosis leading to more high blood pressure. The most important measure that can be taken today to prevent kidney failure is treatment of high blood pressure. The first step in this highly effective treatment is to recognize that high blood pressure exists and to start therapy as soon as possible.

Renal Artery Stenosis

If the problem is a partial blockage of the large artery which brings blood to the kidney (renal artery stenosis), treatment with high blood pressure medicines may not completely control the high blood pressure condition. In fact, this is one of the clues which make doctors think of renal artery stenosis as the underlying cause of high blood pressure. If blood pressure remains high despite an aggressive program of medication, the underlying problem may be a narrowed artery to the kidney. If blood pressure is difficult to control, and if studies document that the cause of high blood pressure is renal artery stenosis, surgery may be indicated. Here the approach will be to remove the narrowed section of the artery so that the blood supply to the kidney is no longer compromised. Blood pressure medication may still be necessary even when the problem with the renal artery is corrected, because there may be small vessel disease as well, and the blood vessels within the kidney are not amenable to surgery. Even if surgery does not fully bring blood pressure down to normal and medication is still necessary, it will usually take less medication to control the blood pressure and the medication that is required will be more effective.

Remember that kidneys that have an impaired blood supply may suffer from loss of function. Sometimes, even if medicines are fully able to control the high blood pressure condition caused by renal artery stenosis, surgery may be recommended. If tests show that the kidneys are gradually losing their ability to filter and purify the blood satisfactorily, it still may be desirable to surgically correct the narrowed renal artery. In this case the reason for surgery is not to control blood pressure—medicines are doing this—but to protect the kidney tissues themselves from progressive loss of function. This is one of the reasons your doctor periodically checks your kidney function while you are being treated for high blood pressure. It is easy to monitor kidney function. All that is required is a small tube of blood so that the BUN and creatinine (see page 38) levels can be measured. If, over a period of time, there is an apparent rise in these numbers, this may indicate that the kidneys have lost some of their ability to filter out the BUN and the creatinine (chemicals which are normally present in low amounts in the bloodstream), and that a progressive loss of normal kidney tissue is occurring. If further investigation demonstrates that renal artery stenosis exists, then it may be possible to prevent further loss of kidney function by operating on the renal artery.

Although the treatment of choice for renal artery stenosis is surgery, this may not always be practical. This is major surgery, and other medical conditions may make it risky for someone to undergo the procedure. Furthermore, surgery may not be desirable even if an individual is a good surgical risk. Atherosclerosis is one of the major causes of obstruction to a major artery to the kidney. If there is atherosclerosis in the major artery, there is a high likelihood that it is present in small arteries of the kidney as well. Fixing the major artery may not work, because the problem with the small arteries remains and can progress.

You can see that it is important that your doctor make a correct diagnosis. If you have high blood pressure due to a narrowed major artery to the kidney, if there is a good chance that the small vessels within your kidney are normal, and if you are a good surgical risk, then your doctor will probably recommend that your high blood pressure condition be treated surgically. In fact, in certain individuals it may be possible to "surgically" correct the narrowed section of the artery without actually undergoing an operation! A new technique has been developed to widen a section of an artery which has been narrowed due to the buildup of cholesterol and deposits of fat within its walls. It was initially employed to widen blood vessels in the legs, but now it is being used to correct narrowed blood vessels in other areas of the body. The technique is called *percutaneous transluminal angioplasty*. In this technique, an instrument is advanced into the artery and then a small balloon is inflated at the site of the narrowing. The pressure exerted by the balloon forces the narrowed section to widen. This technique avoids surgery, because the instrument is advanced into the artery by way of a needle. The needle penetrates the skin and then the instrument is introduced into the artery through the needle and guided to the site of the narrowing. Thus its name: "percutaneous" means through the skin; the inside of an artery is called its "lumen," and "transluminal" means "within the artery"; angioplasty means "repair of a blood vessel." Percutaneous transluminal angioplasty: through the skin and inside the artery approach to repairing a narrowed blood vessel. This is a highly specialized new technique and is not without serious complications. However, it will save an occasional individual who has renal artery stenosis from the need to undergo major surgery.

The first step in arriving at a correct diagnosis is to recognize that there may be some kind of underlying kidney problem which has produced hypertension. This is based upon clues obtained from the medical evaluation of high blood pressure. The next step is to perform an IVP. This X-ray test will strengthen the evidence and allow your doctor to decide whether or not it is worthwhile to proceed with further tests. If the IVP is normal, this means that the clues which suggested underlying kidney disease were probably false. If the IVP is abnormal, this means that the search for a surgically correctable form of hypertension should proceed.

Possible Indications of Underlying Renal Artery Stenosis
Clues from the medical interview: 1. The age at which you were first detected to have high blood pressure. If you were (or are) under 25

years of age (some experts believe this should be under 30 years of age) when you first learned that you have high blood pressure, you may have a problem with one or both kidneys. This is especially true if there is no strong history of high blood pressure in other members of your family. If you were (or are) over 50 years of age when you were first told that you have high blood pressure *and* you know that you did not have high blood pressure before the age of 50, this is also a clue that the kidneys may be the source of the problem. Between the ages of 25 to 50 years of age is when the majority of individuals who have high blood pressure develop essential hypertension. If you were able to live 50 years with a normal blood pressure and suddenly develop high blood pressure, then something may have happened to one or both of your kidneys to have caused its onset. If you are over 50 years of age and have had only mild elevation of blood pressure which suddenly becomes much higher, this might also implicate the kidneys.

2. High blood pressure which has been difficult to control with medicine. Usually, high blood pressure is easily controlled by medicine. If an aggressive program of medication does not fully control high blood pressure, this may indicate that the renal artery is narrowed.

3. An accident which may have injured a kidney. A severe blow to the flank or to the abdomen may damage the kidney and cause high blood pressure.

Clues from the physical examination: 1. A noise heard over the flank or the abdomen. If the major artery which brings blood to the kidney is narrowed for any reason, your doctor may be able to hear a noise over the kidney area when listening with the stethoscope. The major artery to the kidney is large and it carries a great deal of rapidly flowing blood to the kidney. A partial blockage of the artery may be thought of as a rock in a rapidly flowing stream. The rock creates turbulance, and the noise of this turbulant flow can be heard in about 80 percent of the cases of partial obstruction of the renal artery.

2. Abnormal blood vessels (retinal arteries) in the back of your eye. Abnormal retinal arteries reflect poorly controlled blood pressure, and this poor control may be due to renal artery stenosis.

Clues from the laboratory examination: 1. An abnormal urinalysis. The presence of protein in the urine can easily be detected by a simple chemical test. If the kidneys leak protein, this may indicate damage to kidney tissue from a compromised blood supply.

2. High BUN and creatinine. The BUN and the creatinine are relatively simple blood tests which are indicators of how effectively the kidneys filter the blood. Usually these chemicals are rapidly removed from the blood and eliminated in the urine. If they build up to abnormally high levels in the blood, this indicates that

the kidneys are not filtering the blood as well as they should for any one of a number of reasons. One important reason may be loss of tissue because of an inadequate supply of blood.

If your doctor's detective work has produced sufficient evidence to suggest that one or both of your kidneys may be guilty of raising your blood pressure, and especially if the clues point to an obstruction of the renal artery, the next step is to order a rapid-sequence IVP.

The Rapid-Sequence IVP (Intravenous Pyelogram) The kidneys filter and purify the blood. If unwanted chemicals are in the blood, the body may rely upon the kidneys to eliminate them. It is possible to get a good idea of the quality of the kidneys' blood supply by utilizing the kidneys' abilities to eliminate unwanted chemicals from the bloodstream. This is the principle behind the IVP. If the kidney is intact and the major artery to the kidney is free from obstruction, the kidney can remove a chemical from the bloodstream very rapidly. If either the kidney itself is damaged or there is an obstruction to the flow of blood to the kidney, it will take longer to remove an unwanted chemical from the blood and eliminate it in the urine.

The IVP is an X-ray test. A special X-ray dye is injected into a vein in the forearm. This dye is a chemical, which is very rapidly and completely removed from the bloodstream by the kidneys and eliminated in the urine. Usually the kidneys cannot be seen when an X-ray is taken of the abdomen. However, when the kidneys collect and concentrate this X-ray chemical from the bloodstream, the presence of the dye within the kidneys allows them to be seen. After from 10 to 40 minutes, the dye is drained from the kidneys and is stored in the bladder. When this happens, the kidneys can no longer be seen on the X-rays, but the bladder will now be visible.

You have two kidneys. Suppose that the major artery that brings blood to one kidney is normal and that the artery to the other kidney is partially blocked. An X-ray dye is rapidly injected into a vein in your forearm, and a series of X-rays are immediately taken of your abdomen. What will the IVP reveal? Since the dye gets to the kidney with the normal artery first, the first X-ray pictures will show only one kidney. Later, the blood will also get to the kidney with the damaged blood supply, and the later X-rays will show both kidneys. This finding that dye is taken up more rapidly by one kidney than the other is evidence suggesting that the blood supply of one is normal and the blood supply of the other is reduced. It is a *comparison test.*

If the arteries to both kidneys have obstructions within

them, the rapid-sequence IVP is less helpful. All that is known in this case is that both kidneys take up the dye too slowly. Is it because there is narrowing of both renal arteries (which is not common) or because there is damage to the small arteries within both kidneys (which is common)?

The rapid-sequence IVP study cannot *prove* that there is a partial obstruction of a major artery: it can only *suggest* it. The problem may be within the kidney. The test, however, does allow your doctor to decide whether or not it is worthwhile to proceed with further diagnostic studies.

It is not necessary to be hospitalized to have the IVP. It takes about 90 minutes to complete. The only discomfort it produces is a brief uncomfortably warm sensation immediately upon injection of the dye into the vein in your forearm. The test is generally quite safe. Rarely, an individual can develop a serious allergic-type reaction to the dye and this is a potential hazard. If you know that you have had a reaction to an X-ray dye before, or if you have a history of allergy to shellfish or iodides, it is important that you let your doctor know this. You must also tell the doctors and technicians who perform the X-rays. The IVP can usually still be performed safely, but you may be given medications before you receive the X-ray dye to prevent a reaction. Safe and effective medications are available which usually will protect you from a reaction even if you have had a reaction to the dye in the past.

If you have diabetes mellitus (sugar diabetes) do NOT have an IVP until you have extensively discussed the need for it with your doctor. For unknown reasons, individuals with diabetes mellitus may experience a serious and sometimes permanent amount of damage to the kidneys when they undergo the IVP test. The information gained from the IVP may or may not warrant this risk. This is something you and your doctor will have to decide. You now have enough information about high blood pressure and its causes to share in this decision, and your doctor will be happy that you wish to participate.

If the rapid-sequence IVP suggests that the blood supply to one kidney is normal but the blood supply to the other kidney is impaired, it is still not clear whether the problem lies in the major artery to the kidney or within the kidney itself. It is critical to know this in order to decide whether you can benefit from surgery. This information will be obtained by an arteriogram. This is a sophisticated study of blood vessels which must be performed in the hospital.

Suppose the rapid-sequence IVP suggests that the blood supply to *both kidneys* is abnormal. Should the arteriogram be done? Probably not. Here is where the clues from the medical evaluation of high blood pressure again become valuable. If you are under 25 (or 30) and have no strong family history of high blood pressure or any prior history of serious kidney diseases such as nephritis, then you may be one of the rare individuals who was born with congenital narrowing of both renal arteries. With this historical information, it may be worthwhile to go ahead with the arteriogram. If you are over 50 years of age and know that your blood pressure was previously normal and have this IVP result, then you may benefit from the arteriogram. In most other instances, it is not worthwhile proceeding with further diagnostic tests. In most instances, this IVP result indicates that the damage is within the kidneys. Surgery is not helpful in such cases. The arteriogram should be performed only if there is a good possibility that a surgically correctable obstruction of both renal arteries will be discovered.

The Arteriogram   The direct study of arteries by X-ray is called arteriography. An arteriogram is an X-ray study of an artery. The test is performed by introducing a small plastic tube into the body and positioning it near the opening of the artery which is to be studied. An X-ray dye is then rapidly injected into the artery, and an X-ray movie is taken. This allows the progress of the dye to be followed as it flows along the course of the artery. An X-ray movie is not much different from the movies that you are accustomed to viewing, and it is viewed much the same way. The X-ray film is developed and projected upon a screen. This allows for significant magnification and the blood vessels are seen in great detail by this technique. If an artery is obstructed, there will be no question about it.

To understand the technique employed to X-ray the arteries that provide blood to the kidneys, you need to know a little basic anatomy. The major artery which takes blood away from the heart is called the aorta. In the chest, branches come off the aorta to supply blood to the head and to the arms. The aorta then continues into the abdomen, where blood vessels branch off to supply the organs within the abdomen. The two arteries to the kidneys (the renal arteries) branch off the aorta in the upper part of the abdomen. When the aorta reaches the bottom of the abdomen it divides in two and continues into the legs. You can easily feel the pulse of the major artery to each leg by pressing with your fingers on the inner part of your groin.

A renal arteriogram is performed by introducing a small plastic tube into the artery at the level of the groin and threading it back up the aorta until the tube is at the level of the kidneys. This X-ray examination is not difficult to perform, and the major discomfort occurs when the tube is introduced into the artery at the groin. This discomfort is reduced by first injecting a local an-

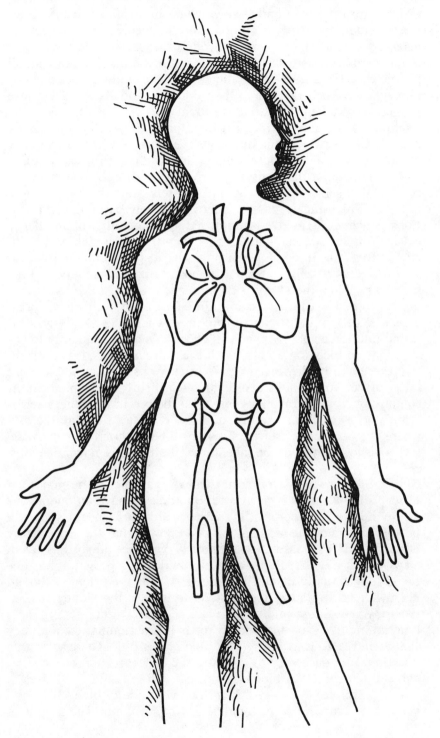

The aorta and major arteries

esthetic into the skin and tissues which lie over the artery. Once the area over the artery is numb, a special needle is placed into the artery, a wire is then inserted through the needle, and the needle is removed. The wire serves as a guide for the insertion of a small plastic tube. This tube is threaded up the aorta until it reaches the kidney area. An X-ray dye is then injected, and X-ray movies are immediately taken of the kidney area. The picture will show the anatomy of the arteries in great detail, and they will immediately provide the answer to the questions, "Is it renal artery stenosis or small vessel disease?" Both kidneys are studied at the same time.

The major discomfort experienced during the test is an uncomfortable sensation of heat immediately after the X-ray dye is injected. This quickly passes. There are a few possible complications. Since an X-ray dye is employed, the possibility of an allergy exists. You already know about this from the discussion of the IVP above. Bleeding into the groin after the test is completed is also possible. This is why you must be hospitalized to undergo an arteriogram. After the study is completed, you will have to remain quietly in bed until the next morning. For much of this time, pressure will be applied to your groin area where the needle was inserted into the artery. Nurses will check this area frequently to ensure that no bleeding occurs. With these precautions, it is unlikely that there will be any bleeding. To further ensure that no bleeding takes place, you should avoid taking aspirin or any medication containing aspirin for about one week before having the arteriogram performed. Very rarely, a blood clot can form at the site where the tube was inserted. This is called an *arterial thrombosis*. If this occurs, steps will be taken immediately to remove the blood clot.

Suppose the arteriogram shows that one of the major arteries to the kidneys is narrowed. Should you have an operation? You will have to undergo still another test before this question can be answered. For the moment, all you know is that the renal artery is narrowed. You assume this means that the kidney has taken steps which have resulted in an elevated blood pressure, but has the kidney actually taken these steps? Maybe the artery, although narrowed, still allows enough blood to flow to the kidney to keep it happy. You must find out how this kidney is functioning. Is it functioning like a normal kidney, or is it functioning like a kidney that believes it must raise the blood pressure? To answer this question, it is necessary to measure the concentration of a chemical called *renin* in the bloodstream.

"Simple," you say. "Just take a sample of blood from the vein in my arm and do the analysis." Not so simple. The sample of blood must be taken directly from the vein that drains the kidney. Thus, another tube!

The Renal Vein Renin Test When a reduction in the blood supply to a kidney is interpreted by the kidney to mean that there is a need for it to raise the blood pressure, it responds to this perceived threat to the body by making a chemical called *renin*. Renin is released into the veins that drain the kidney, and it starts up the chain of events which results in the retention of salt and water. This is how the kidney goes about raising the blood pressure.

You know that the kidney has a narrowed artery because you saw it on the X-ray study. Now, you need to know if this narrowed artery is causing the kidney to raise the blood pressure. If it is, the renin level in the vein draining the kidney will be abnormally high. It is not sufficient just to take a sample of blood from the vein in your arm and measure the renin level. Even if it is very high, there is not complete assurance that the renin comes from the suspected kidney. It might be coming from the kidney which you believe to be normal. Not likely, but possible. Since we are talking about major surgery, guessing is not allowed.

The final study which must be performed to prove that the suspected kidney is truly raising the blood pressure is the *renal vein renin test*. To perform this test, a tube must be placed into the renal vein. This is done by a technique quite similar to that of the renal arteriogram and can be done at the same time. Instead of placing the small plastic tube into the artery in the groin, the tube is introduced into the vein. It is threaded up to the level of the kidneys and placed into first one renal vein and then the other. Samples of blood are taken from each kidney and sent to the laboratory for analysis. A sample of blood is also taken from a vein elsewhere in the body, so that the renin level in the vein draining each kidney can be compared to the renin level of the rest of the body. If one kidney is normal and one is making too much renin, the laboratory will confirm this by reporting too much renin in one vein and the same amount of renin in the other vein as in the rest of the body. (Since the abnormal kidney is producing too much renin, the normal kidney can rest; it has no reason to make renin at all, so its renin level simply reflects the level of renin in the rest of the body. If both kidneys have a problem with their blood supply, the renin level will be high in both samples.) With this information, a decision can now be confidently made about the cause of your high blood pressure. You now have assurance that the narrowing of the renal artery is the underlying cause.

There are few complications associated with renal vein renin test. It is just a more sophisticated way of taking a blood sample. There is some mild discomfort in the groin area where the tube is inserted, but that is the extent of it. Some X-ray dye is injected to identify the opening of veins draining each kidney, so the same potential problem of an allergic reaction exists as previously discussed. Many medications can interfere with the renin test. It is generally recommended that you stop all blood pressure medicines one to two weeks before you undergo this test. If your blood pressure is seriously high it may not be safe to stop blood pressure medicines even for this relatively brief period of time. Since certain of the blood pressure medicines do not interfere with the renin test, your doctor can switch you to one of these if necessary.

It is important to emphasize that even though there is clear evidence that renal artery stenosis is the cause of high blood pressure, surgical correction may not be desirable. If the narrowing is due to atherosclerosis, surgery may be only temporarily successful. Atherosclerosis is usually a progressive disease, and it affects large arteries as well as small ones. If there is good reason to suspect that the kidney's blood supply will in any event be threatened because of progressive atherosclerosis, then the risk of the surgical procedure may not be warranted.

At times, a kidney will be so extensively damaged by the combination of inadequate blood supply and high blood pressure that it becomes small and nonfunctioning. Should it be surgically removed in this case? If the high blood pressure cannot be well controlled with medicines, and if the tests prove that this shrunken kidney is producing an excessive amount of renin, then such surgery is indicated. Since one kidney has already been lost, it becomes imperative to do everything possible to preserve the function of the other kidney. One of the most important measures that your doctor can take to preserve your kidney function is to ensure that your blood pressure is under good control at all times. If medicines can't accomplish this, then removal of the kidney is probably indicated. High blood pressure medicines may still be required, but once the seriously damaged kidney has been removed, it should be possible to bring blood pressure down to normal and keep it there with fewer medicines and with a less complicated program.

You can see that there is a lot that has to be accomplished before a decision can be made to operate on the major artery to a kidney to treat high blood pressure. Fortunately, it is only necessary to proceed with the more complicated tests if the rapid-sequence IVP is abnormal. Since the IVP can be performed without the need of hospitalization, your doctor should find it necessary to hospitalize you only when there is very strong evidence to suggest that your blood pressure problem is due to a narrowing of one or both renal arteries.

HYPERALDOSTERONISM

The adrenal glands produce many important hormones that regulate chemical metabolism. One of these hormones is *aldosterone.* Aldosterone is a hormone which helps the body retain salt.

Your body has various ways of controlling the amount of salt and water that it needs. One method of regulation is thirst. If you need water, a center in the brain senses that you are becoming dehydrated and sends out a message which causes you to drink more water. Another regulatory mechanism is blood pressure. If your kidneys sense that the blood pressure is dropping too low, they start their machinery going to retain salt and water. Your adrenal glands also get into the act. When there is a need for the body to retain salt and water, the adrenal glands release the hormone aldosterone into the bloodstream. This hormone has a powerful effect on the kidneys, and it forces them to retain salt and water. Occasionally one or both of the adrenal glands will become overactive and produce too much aldosterone. As a result, the kidney retains too much salt and water, and this, as you know, results in high blood pressure. This unusual hormonal condition is called *hyperaldosteronism,* and sometimes it can be corrected by surgery. (A word about medical language. "Hyper" means "too much." "Ism" means "condition." Hyperaldosteronism can be translated, "condition of too much aldosterone.")

Possible Indicators of Hyperaldosteronism

Clues from the physical examination: There are no helpful clues from the physical examination.

Clues from the laboratory examination: Abnormally low blood potassium. If the adrenal gland is producing so much aldosterone that the blood pressure becomes too high, the level of blood potassium will be too low. If your doctor finds that you have high blood pressure *and* that your potassium level is persistently low, this is a clue to consider this rare abnormality of adrenal gland function. You will remember from Chapter 7 that diuretics characteristically produce a low potassium. Consequently, this clue is *not* valid if you were taking a diuretic at the time that the blood sample was taken for potassium analysis. You must stop the diuretic for about one week and then have your blood tested again. When it is clear that the persistently low blood potassium is not the result of a diuretic, there is good reason for your doctor to suspect that you may have hyperaldosteronism.

Once there is information about your blood potassium level to suggest the presence of this abnormality of adrenal gland function, one further blood test can be done in your doctor's office to support this clue. This test is called the *blood renin level*. This is the same chemical, renin, mentioned before. This time, a simple measure of the concentration of renin in a blood sample taken from a vein in your arm is sufficient. It is not necessary to be in the hospital, and it is not necessary to place tubes within the body.

Why is it helpful to know the concentration of renin in the bloodstream? You will remember that when the kidneys wish to raise the blood pressure, the first thing they do is release renin into the bloodstream. High blood pressure due to kidney diseases means high blood renin. In the case of hyperaldosteronism, the adrenal gland, by overproducing aldosterone hormone, is forcing the kidneys to retain salt and water. Since the blood pressure is going to be too high anyway, there is no reason for the kidneys to secrete renin to make the blood pressure any higher. Therefore the kidneys stop making renin. This may help prevent the pressure from getting too high. Thus if you have high blood pressure, a low potassium, *and* a low blood renin, the evidence to suggest that you have hyperaldosteronism is very strong.

To prove the diagnosis, you may have to be hospitalized so that you can undergo careful tests to analyze the function of your adrenal gland. These tests are called *endocrine* tests. The *endocrine glands* are the glands which make hormones. An *endocrinologist* is a medical specialist who is expert in the metabolism of the endocrine glands. Tests of endocrine metabolism are seldom uncomfortable. They are simply a series of blood and urine tests performed under special conditions. Ordering the proper sequence of tests and properly interpreting the results of these tests requires a specialist, and your doctor will want to obtain the guidance of an endocrinologist at this point of the investigation.

Testing a gland to determine whether it is making too much or too little of a hormone is more complicated than you might think. You might reasonably assume that if the purpose of the investigation is to find out whether or not there is too much of the hormone aldosterone in the bloodstream, all that is required is a sample of blood. Why can't the endocrinologist just take a sample of blood and analyze it? Doesn't too much aldosterone mean an overactive gland?

It is not that simple. Glands that produce hormones can be thought of as a series of traffic islands located along a highway to regulate the flow of traffic. The traffic lights of each traffic island do not work in isolation. Each works in cooperation with the lights of the traffic island coming before it and one coming after it. They all work together to regulate the flow of automobiles coming down the highway. A driver may believe that the traffic lights of one particular island are much too slow. Is this true? The only way to be sure is to know what is happening to the traffic in front and in back of the car. Maybe the traffic in front has become so congested that a message came to this traffic island to tell it to slow down the flow of traffic so that the congestion further down the highway can be cleared.

Glands that produce hormones are like a series of traffic islands. They are located in various areas of the body, and they all work together to regulate metabolism. If one gland seems to be overactive, is it because it is responding to a signal from another gland, or has something happened to its own "wiring" which has caused it to become independent of the other glands? If the adrenal gland is producing too much aldosterone, is this because the adrenal gland received a message from one of the other "traffic islands" telling it to do this (in which case the gland is working appropriately) or has the adrenal gland decided to take off on its own and inappropriately produce too much hormone? In one case, the problem lies not within the adrenal gland but with some other part of the system, the part which is giving the message to the adrenal gland. In the other case, the problem lies with the adrenal gland itself. Deciding which situation exists is the job of the endocrinologist. It is necessary not only to measure the concentration of the hormone itself, but also to measure the concentration of *the messengers* which tell the gland what to do. The complicated part of the study of metabolism is the analysis of the messengers.

An analysis of metabolism must be carried out under very exacting conditions. For this reason, hospitalization is often required. The nature of your diet, the quantity and types of liquids you drink, and the timing of your blood and urine tests all must be precisely controlled. It will take about a week of sequential blood and urine tests to finally determine whether the reason you produce too much aldosterone is the independent and inappropriate overactivity of the adrenal gland or a malfunction in some other part of the traffic regulation system.

Once it has been decided that it is the adrenal gland itself which is at fault, the problem is still not completely solved. You have two adrenal glands. Is only one overactive or are both overactive? This is a critical decision, because surgery usually will correct your high blood pressure if only one gland is overactive, but it will not correct the condition if both glands are overactive. X-ray tests and more sophisticated blood sampling techniques are required to answer this question.

If a gland is overactive, it usually becomes abnormally large. One way of deciding whether one or both adrenal glands are overactive is to find out if both glands are unusually large or if only one gland is enlarged. Two special types of X-ray tests can provide this information. One text is called a *nuclear scan*, and the other is called a *C.A.T. scan*.

Nuclear scans are performed by injection of a tiny quantity of radioactive chemical into the bloodstream and taking pictures of the radioactivity. The amount of radioactivity is extremely small, about the same amount as or less than you receive during an ordinary X-ray examination. These tests are entirely safe. Unlike the IVP or arteriogram, there is no danger of an allergic-type reaction, and this is another attractive feature of this type of diagnostic test. The radioactive chemical must be specially designed to be removed from the bloodstream by the gland which it is desired to study. If only this gland takes up the radioactivity from the bloodstream, the radioactivity will all be concentrated in that small area of the body. A picture of the radioactivity can then be taken, and the picture will have the shape either of the entire gland or of that part of the gland where the radioactive chemical is concentrated. The thyroid gland, for example, selectively metabolizes iodine. If it is desired to take a picture of the thyroid gland, a small amount of radioactive iodine can be given and pictures taken of the neck. Once the radioactive iodine has been concentrated in the thyroid gland, the pictures will clearly show the gland.

The C.A.T. scan is a way of taking X-rays that has proven to be a powerful new diagnostic technique. "C.A.T." means "computer axial tomography." It combines an X-ray machine with a computer. Instead of an X-ray picture being developed on a photographic plate, the X-ray signals are fed into a computer. You have probably had X-ray pictures taken, so you know that usually the technique is much like regular photography. A camera uses visible light waves to develop your picture on photographic film. An X-ray camera uses X-ray waves to develop your picture on X-ray film. The X-rays are shorter and have more energy than visible light rays, and they are able to penetrate the body and allow pictures to be taken of internal structures. Most X-ray pictures are taken from a single angle, the same way that a photograph is taken.

The computer is an extraordinarily powerful analytical tool, and it allows an X-ray picture to be taken in an entirely new way. Instead of a picture of internal structures being taken from just one angle the way an ordinary X-ray is taken, the picture is taken from many angles and each picture is stored in the computer rather than developed on X-ray film. A circle has 360 degrees, and in essence 360 photographs are taken and fed into the computer. The computer then assembles all the information to form a single picture which shows the internal structures with amazing detail. However, this picture is entirely different from the usual X-ray picture. A regular X-ray will show an entire structure—for example, the entire lungs from top to bottom. Like a regular photograph, such a picture is flat and lacks the dimension of depth. Since a C.A.T. picture is taken by circling completely around the lungs, it has depth, but it gives a picture of only one plane of the lungs. For example, if the X-ray beam was circled around the chest at the level of the nipples, the computer picture will show a detailed view of the lungs only at that level. The picture will have depth, but will lack length. To see the whole lung, an entire series of pictures of the chest must be taken, starting at the top of the chest and going down to the bottom of the chest. Instead of having a single picture of your lungs, your doctor will have perhaps 20 or 30 pictures, each depicting "one slice" through the chest cavity. Each slice shows everything that is in the chest cavity at that one level. The name reflects this "slice" effect. "Axial" means "the line about which a rotating body turns." In this case the axis is an imaginary line through the center of your body around which the X-ray camera rotates. "Tomography" means "X-ray photography of a selected plane of the body." Computer axial tomography: assisted X-ray computer photography taken by rotating (an X-ray beam) around a central point within the body.

A C.A.T. scan of your abdomen allows your doctor to see the anatomy of the organs within the abdomen with great clarity. Both adrenal glands can be seen by this revolutionary new X-ray technique. If one or both of the adrenal glands are enlarged, this may be an indication that one or both of the glands are overactive.

To confirm the result of the C.A.T. and nuclear scans, a small tube is placed into the vein in the groin and threaded up to the level of the adrenal glands. A sample of blood is then taken from each gland. The gland which is thought to be overactive should have an abnormally high level of aldosterone coming from the vein which drains it. It is necessary to use a small amount of X-ray dye to perform this test. The dye is necessary to identify the opening of the veins, so there is the possibility of an allergic reaction to the dye.

While the plastic tube is in the adrenal vein, it is possible to inject X-ray dye under pressure and take an X-ray picture of the adrenal vein. The dye is forced up into the gland, and an X-ray picture is immediately taken while the dye is concentrated in the gland. Taking a picture of the gland by utilizing its vein is called *venography*, and the test itself is called a *venogram*. This test is potentially hazardous. The adrenal gland is fragile, and forcing the dye up into it under pressure occasionally causes the gland to bleed. This, in turn, can lead to permanent damage. Of course, there is also the usual problem of possible allergy to the X-ray dye.

If all these tests confirm that only one gland is overactive, surgery usually will cure the high blood pressure condition. If both glands are found to be overactive, surgery will not work, but medicine will usually successfully control the blood pressure condition. Although medicine will successfully bring the blood pressure down to normal and keep it there, you cannot call it a cure because the high blood pressure condition will return if the medicine is stopped. Even though surgery will cure the high blood pressure condition when only one gland is enlarged, it is not absolutely necessary to undergo this major surgical procedure. Usually, the condition can be treated with medicine, but the medicine must be taken for the rest of one's life. Only if the medicine is poorly tolerated or causes too many side effects is it necessary to proceed with surgery.

The potassium-sparing agent spironolactone will successfully control the high blood pressure caused by the overproduction of aldosterone by one or both adrenal glands. The important features of spironolactone were outlined in Chapter 8. You already know that the hormone aldosterone works by forcing the kidney to retain salt and water. Spironolactone has the unique ability to prevent aldosterone from working. This medication acts like a fence, protecting the kidneys from aldosterone. It is a very effective medicine in the treatment of hyperaldosteronism, but it has to be given in much larger amounts than described in Chapter 8. To build a big enough fence around the kidneys to protect them from the abnormally high concentration of aldosterone, 200 or 300 mg of spironolactone may be required per day. The more that is used, the more likely it is that side effects will occur. Men especially may find it difficult to tolerate this high level of the medicine because of the uncomfortable side effect of enlarged and tender breasts. The possible menstrual irregularity it causes in women may be better tolerated. The side effects of spironolactone can be reduced by adding other high blood pressure medicines so that a lower dosage of spironolactone can be taken. Often, one of the thiazide diuretics discussed in Chapter 7 is employed. If only one gland is overactive and the side effects are not well tolerated, surgery is an alternative. If both glands are overactive, it will be necessary to put up with the side effects.

CUSHING'S DISEASE

Cushing's disease is another rare abnormality of adrenal gland function which causes high blood pressure. The adrenal gland produces many important hormones. We have just discussed aldosterone, which helps regulate salt metabolism. Another very important adrenal gland hormone is *hydrocortisone* or *cortisol*. Hydrocortisone regulates many aspects of the body's metabolism. It helps regulate the way the body fights infection and allergies, plays a role in sugar and fat metabolism, and helps regulate the growth and quality of bone, elastic tissue, and skin. Because hydrocortisone has so many important functions, its overproduction by the adrenal glands, Cushing's disease, is very dramatic in its effects upon the body. There are many prominent clues which suggest the overproduction of cortisone, and high blood pressure is one of the least dramatic of these clues.

Possible Indications of Cushing's Disease

Clues from the medical interview: 1. Change in appearance. The overproduction of cortisone causes excess fatty tissues to be deposited in three characteristic areas of the body: the face, the back of the neck, and the abdomen. The face becomes quite rounded and full; a prominent lump of fat appears on the back of the neck; the abdomen becomes fat.

2. Weight gain. This is to be expected since there is excess formation of fat.

3. Fatigue and weakness. These are not reliable symptoms since they occur so commonly with other diseases and also appear when there is anxiety or depression.

4. Skin changes. Woman may notice increased facial hair. Both men and women may notice purple or violet colored stretch marks on the skin, especially about the abdomen. Although stretch marks are common when any weight gain occurs, the characteristic color helps to distinguish the stretch marks of overproduction of cortisone from the stretch marks of simple obesity. Occasionally, both men and women may notice that their skin is getting darker. Acne may suddenly appear in someone who never had acne before. If someone already has acne, it may become worse.

5. Cessation of menstruation. Women who suffer from overproduction of cortisone often stop having periods.

6. Personality changes. For some reason, individuals who have too much cortisone in their system may undergo a personality change. Sometimes this is dramatic. The usual change is an increased irritability and a tendency to have rapid and sudden changes in emotion.

Clues from the physical examination: 1. Body appearance. As might be expected, the changes in body appearance will be obvious to the physician. Of course, the accumulation of fat in the face, back of the neck, and abdomen is not unique to overproduction of cortisone. This can happen with ordinary weight gain as well. Your own observation that these changes are recent will help your doctor. The typical color of the stretch marks will also help in this regard. Excess hair production in women is usually a family trait. If your doctor notices excess hair, you will be questioned about whether your mother, your sisters, or your aunts have a similar problem. The distribution of fat in the face, back of the neck, and abdomen in association with the typical colored stretch marks and excess body hair often presents a very characteristic appearance. The typical skin changes of acne may also be present.

Clues from the laboratory examination: 1. Abnormally high blood sugar. Excess hydrocortisone production almost always produces a tendency to diabetes mellitus. In fact, sometimes the sugar rises to such high levels that treatment with insulin or an oral diabetic medication is required.

The findings of high blood pressure, characteristic obesity, high blood sugar, and abnormal skin changes, along with the clues from the medical interview all present at the same time suggest that you may suffer from Cushing's disease. It is very important to remember that obese individuals commonly have high blood pressure and also commonly have a high blood sugar. The distribution of the fatty tissue should be typical. Stretch marks should have the typical violet or purple color. Your observations that you have experienced some change in personality or emotions, or that you have experienced irregular or absent menstrual periods are important. No one abnormality is particularly helpful. Clues must be present from all three parts of the medical evaluation.

If clues are present from the medical interview, the physical examination, and the basic laboratory examination, your doctor may wish to further explore the possibility of your having this rare condition. Further studies are best performed in the hospital under the guidance of an endocrinologist. It will be necessary to carry out tests of your metabolism to prove that there is excess production of cortisone and to find out what has happened to cause this to occur. Are one or both adrenal glands independently making too much cortisone? Or are the glands being forced to make too much hormone by the overactivity of another gland? The tests that are required to answer these questions are not particularly uncomfortable, but they require expert knowledge of glandular metabolism, and your doctor will require the expert guidance of the endocrinologist to arrange the appropriate blood and urine tests and to assist in the interpretation of the test results.

Hydrocortisone is produced by the adrenal glands, which are located in the abdomen just above the level of the kidneys. In the normal individual, the production of cortisone by the adrenal gland is regulated by a messenger hormone called *ACTH*. ACTH is produced by a special part of the brain called the *pituitary gland*. It enters the bloodstream and goes to the adrenal glands. ACTH is the pituitary gland's messenger to the adrenals; it brings the message, "Make more hydrocortisone." When cortisone production is too high, it may be because the pituitary gland is sending too many ACTH messages, or it may be because one or both adrenal glands have become independently overactive. On rare occasions, ACTH may be produced not by the pituitary gland but by a lung cancer or some other abnormal growth of tissue within the body; the abnormal tissue behaves like the pituitary gland and has the ability to make ACTH in large amounts.

The first tests performed in the hospital will be a series of blood and urine tests to prove that you really do produce hydrocortisone in excessive amounts. Then tests will be performed to determine whether the problem is due to an overactive pituitary gland which is making too much ACTH, or whether there is an unusual growth within the body which is producing too much ACTH, or whether the problem is due to the independent overactivity of one or both adrenal glands. If the adrenal gland is at fault, it must be determined whether one or both glands are overactive. This is accomplished by using the nuclear scan, C.A.T. scan, and arteriography techniques that were outlined earlier in this chapter.

Cushing's disease is a serious disease. Fortunately it is rare. It can be corrected only by removing the source of excessive hydrocortisone production. This may mean operating on the pituitary gland or decreasing the activity of the pituitary gland by X-ray treatments. It may mean removing one adrenal gland. It may mean removing both adrenal glands. It may mean removing a lung cancer or some other tumorous growth. All these are major operations, and all must be performed by expert surgeons with much experience.

PHEOCHROMOCYTOMA

Pheochromocytoma is a rare condition of the nervous system which characteristically causes high blood pressure. The chemical messenger norepinephrine was described in Chapters 5 and 6. To briefly review: The nervous system is a major regulator of the blood pressure machines, and norepinephrine is a chemical messenger of the nervous system. It gives the message, "Raise the blood pressure," to the blood pressure regulating machines. Rarely, one part of the nervous system will begin manufacturing too much norepinephrine, and this causes high blood pressure. The production of norepinephrine occurs in a special area of the nervous system called the *sympathetic ganglia*. When some of the sympathetic ganglia become overactive and secrete too much norepinephrine, this portion of the nervous system is called a *pheochromocytoma*.

Possible Indications of Pheochromocytoma

Clues from the medical interview: 1. Weight loss. Individuals with pheochromocytoma tend to lose weight.

2. Other members of the family having had glandular tumors. Rarely, in some families there is an inherited predisposition to certain glandular tumors, especially tumors of the thyroid and parathyroid glands. For some reason, pheochromocytoma occurs more often in individuals whose family members have one of these glandular tumors.

3. Heart palpitations and inappropriately excessive perspiration. Norepinephrine causes the heart to speed up, and it may cause palpitations. Usually, when there is an excessive amount of norepinephrine in the body, there is also an excessive amount of a closely related chemical called *epinephrine*. One clue to the presence of excessive epinephrine is inappropriately excessive sweating.

Clues from the physical examination: There are no really helpful clues from the physical examination.

Clues from the laboratory examination: 1. Abnormally high blood sugar. This is mainly due to epinephrine. When the concentration of norepinephrine is elevated in the body, the concentration of epinephrine usually is also elevated. An excessive amount of either chemical causes the blood sugar level to be abnormally high.

You can see that there are not many clues which suggest the presence of this rare disease. Probably the best clue is the finding of a high blood sugar in a thin person who also has high blood pressure. However, usually this will simply indicate a tendency toward diabetes mellitus and not pheochromocytoma.

Fortunately, it is possible to establish the diagnosis of this unusual high blood pressure condition by ordering a simple urine test which does not require hospitalization.

If there is an overproduction of norepinephrine (and epinephrine) by the nervous system, these chemicals will appear in excess amounts in the urine. If your doctor wishes to explore the possibility that a pheochromocytoma underlies your high blood pressure, you will be requested to collect all of your urine for 24 hours in a special container. The urine will then be analyzed in the laboratory. It is very important for you to know that many medicines can interfere with this chemical analysis. You must report to your doctor all the medicines that you are taking. Usually you will be instructed to stop *all* medicines for a few days before collecting the urine sample. The common cold and sinus and allergy preparations can interfere with the test, as can medications given by psychiatrists to treat anxiety and depression. Some of the medicines given to treat high blood pressure can also interfere, and this is especially true of methyldopa. At one time it was necessary to eat a special diet before and during the urine collection, but this is no longer necessary for most urine tests. However, if your doctor orders the VMA urine test, it will be necessary for you to follow a special diet.

VMA is the chemical abbreviation for a compound (methoxy-4-hydroxymandelic acid) present in abnormally high concentration in the urine of an individual who has a pheochromocytoma. VMA is chemically related to the flavoring agent vanilla which is added to many food products and which occurs naturally in some foods as vanillin. If such foods are eaten shortly before or during the time that urine is collected for VMA assay, a falsely high number can result. To avoid this, coffee, tea, nuts, bananas, cake, ice cream, and any other food which has added vanilla must be eliminated from the diet for about 3 days prior to the urine collection.

If your doctor finds that you do have an abnormal amount of the chemical in your urine, then hospitalization will be necessary to locate the pheochromocytoma. Usually it is in a small section of the nervous system which lies in the abdomen within or near the adrenal gland. Highly sophisticated X-ray techniques will be required, and these may include a C.A.T. scan, arteriography, and venography. These special tests and their potential complications have already been described. Once the source of the excessive production of norepinephrine and epinephrine is located, surgery will be required to remove it. Removal of the pheochromocytoma does not in any way impair the normal function of the nervous system, for this abnormal area is quite small and it is far removed from the spinal cord.

Occasionally surgery cannot be performed. Fortunately, there is a medication available, phenoxybenzamine (Dibenzyline), which will counteract most of the effects of a pheochromocytoma and control the blood pressure, but blood pressure is not as well controlled by this medication as it is by surgery.

COARCTATION OF THE AORTA

This is a rare form of high blood pressure caused by a malformation of the major blood vessel which takes blood away from the heart, the aorta. This congenital abnormality is present at birth, but it may not be discovered until later in life.

The aorta is the major artery which takes blood away from the heart. Arteries first branch from it to supply the head, and then branches come off to supply the arms. The aorta then continues down the body to supply the organs within the abdomen. Finally it divides in two and goes into each leg. Coarctation of the aorta occurs when there is a narrowed section of the aorta. Usually this narrowed section is located just below the branches that leave the aorta to supply the arms. The heart must pump more forcefully to get blood to the organs of the abdomen and legs, for these are supplied with blood from the section of the aorta below the narrowed section. The arteries that come off the aorta *before* it narrows will have a high blood pressure, and the arteries that come off the aorta *after* it narrows will have a low blood pressure. The narrowed section of the aorta is like a pressure valve: on one side of the valve the pressure will be high and on the other side the pressure will be low. Since the blood vessels to the arms branch from the aorta before it narrows, the blood pressure will be abnormally high in the arms. Because the blood vessels to the legs are below the narrowing, the blood pressure in the legs will be low.

Possible Indications of Coarctation of the Aorta
Clues from the medical interview: 1. History of murmur. The narrowed section of the aorta creates a partial obstruction to the flow of blood. The turbulent flow can be heard as a loud blowing sound. You may have been previously told that you have a heart murmur, because sometimes it is difficult to distinguish whether the murmur is arising from the heart itself or from the aorta.

Clues from the physical examination: 1. Abnormal sound. Your doctor will hear the loud blowing sound in your chest.

2. Abnormal distribution of blood pressure. Usually, when an individual has high blood pressure, it is high in both the arms and the legs. When coarctation of the aorta is present, the blood pressure is high in the arms but low in the legs.

Clues from the laboratory examination: 1. Abnormal chest X-ray. The deformed aorta causes a characteristic X-ray picture.

2. Abnormal electrocardiogram. If the deformed aorta has forced the heart to work under too much strain, this may be apparant on the electrocardiogram, a test which provides a permanent record of the heart's pattern of electrical activity. Obtaining an electrocardiogram is a painless procedure which takes only a few minutes to accomplish. Often, the heart's pattern of electrical activity is altered by a health condition, and many health conditions produce patterns which are so characteristic that they can be diagnosed from the electrocardiogram alone.

The diagnosis of coarctation of the aorta is established with near certainty from these findings alone. The treatment of this condition is always surgical. Before the surgeon operates to repair the narrowed section, a detailed picture of its anatomy is required. This is obtained from an arteriogram of this section of the aorta. As you know, the arteriogram is performed by inserting a plastic tube into the groin and threading up to the desired location in the aorta. In some cases an artery in the arm may be used. X-ray dye is then injected, and X-ray movies are taken. The risks and complications of an arteriogram have already been described.

10

IF YOU TAKE THE PILL

The most reliable method of contraception is the oral contraceptive pill. Unfortunately, it is also the method with the most serious cardiovascular side effects. The contraceptive pill is one of the most widely used and one of the best studied medicines in the world. It is estimated that the pill is used by 60 million women worldwide today. In the United States alone, about one woman of every nine between the ages of 15 and 44 takes the pill. That's about 17 million women. In many countries, the number of women who take the pill is much greater than it is in the United States.

Yet, despite its popularity, the use of the pill is on the decline in Western Europe and America. What is the cause of this decline? Why are fewer Western European and American women now using the pill?

The pill is becoming a less popular method of pregnancy prevention because careful studies have clearly demonstrated that it has the potential of causing serious and even fatal illness in those who take it, and an increasing number of women have decided that the risks are too great for the single benefit of contraception. If you have high blood pressure, perhaps you should join the many women who have made this decision. Many doctors would agree that no woman who has high blood pressure should take the pill and no woman who develops high blood pressure while taking the pill should continue to use it.

Here are the facts. The pill raises the blood pressure of almost every woman who takes it. The pill increases your risk of heart attack. The pill increases your risk of stroke, and this risk is not entirely reversed when you stop the pill. The chance of your suffering any of these complications is much greater if you take the pill and also have high blood pressure, or smoke cigarettes, or are overweight, or are over 30 years of age, or have a tendency toward diabetes, or have a high cholesterol number, or have family members with high blood pressure, early heart diseases, or stroke.

Remember that risk factors for heart disease and stroke are additive (see Chapter 4). The pill is a risk factor for heart disease and stroke. High blood pressure is also a risk factor for heart disease and stroke. If you have high blood pressure *and* take the pill, you further increase your chance of having either a heart attack or a stroke. Is the pill worth this risk to you? Once you have a little more detailed information about the potential harm that the contraceptive pills can do to your body, you should have no trouble answering this question.

WHAT IS THE PILL?

You will be better able to understand the discussion of the potentially harmful side effects of the oral contraceptive pill once you understand how the pill works to prevent pregnancy. Most pills are a combination of an *estrogen* and a *progestin*. These are called the "combined" pills. Estrogen and progestin are both female hormones, and they control the menstrual cycle. During the first two weeks of the normal menstrual cycle there is a progressive buildup in the concentration of estrogen in the bloodstream. The estrogen concentration reaches its peak about the fourteenth day. At this point in the cycle, there is a sudden drop in the concentration of estrogen which causes the pituitary gland to release a certain hormone which tells the ovary to release its egg. Once the egg is released, the ovary begins to produce a progestin hormone. The progestin helps prepare the lining of the womb to receive the egg. If the egg does not become fertilized, the concentration of progestin produced by the ovary falls to a low level, and menstruation occurs. The cycle is repeated approximately every 28 days.

If the egg becomes fertilized, the production of the progestin continues in order to keep the lining of the womb suitable for the developing egg. Since there is now an egg implanted in the wall of the womb, the body needs some way of making sure that no more eggs come into the womb. Otherwise, it would be possible to have another egg become fertilized, and this is clearly undesirable. The body solves this problem in a very clever way. At the same time that the progestin works on the lining of the womb to keep it suitable for the egg, it also tells the pituitary gland to stop making the hormone that signals the ovary to release its egg. Because the egg is fertilized, the progestin level does not fall. Because the progestin level does not fall, the pituitary keeps getting the signal to send no more messenger hormone to the ovary. Thus, the ovary stops releasing eggs. A clever and economical system!

Suppose that a woman takes an oral progestin. As far as the pituitary gland is concerned, if the progestin level is up, then a pregnancy is present. The pituitary gland cannot distinguish a progestin which comes in a pill from a progestin which comes from the ovary. Now you know the chemical nature of the first birth control pill and its mechanism of action. The first birth control pill was a progestin. It fools the pituitary gland into thinking that there is a pregnancy present, and in this way it prevents the ovary from releasing any eggs. This form of birth control is called the "progestin only" pill, and it is still in use. Today it is called the *minipill.*

Estrogens also prevent the ovary from releasing its eggs. It was mentioned above that the estrogen concentration peaks at about midcycle and then falls and that the fall in estrogen signals the pituitary to send the hormone messenger to the ovary to tell it to release its egg. If a pill containing estrogen is taken every day, the natural fall in the estrogen level at midcycle is prevented, and the ovary does not receive the signal to release its egg. This is another form of birth control pill, called the "estrogen only" pill. It turns out that a fairly large quantity of estrogen must be taken with this method of birth control, and it is associated with so many undesirable side effects that it is no longer used. (It is still occasionally taken for a few days at a time as the "morning after" pill.)

Thus both estrogen and progestin inhibit the ovary from releasing its eggs. Each hormone works by preventing the pituitary gland from sending its message to release the egg to the ovary. By combining both an estrogen and a progestin into a single pill, it is possible to make an even more effective birth control pill than can be achieved by using only one of the hormones. This form of birth control pill is called the "combined pill." Not only is the combined pill more effective than an estrogen-only pill or a progestin-only pill, but it requires much less estrogen than is contained in an estrogen-only pill. This makes it possible to have an effective birth control pill with far fewer side effects. The majority of contraceptive pills in use today contain both an estrogen and a progestin.

The first combined pills had a relatively high concentration of estrogen, about 100 micrograms. When it was realized that many of the harmful cardiovascular side effects of the contraceptive pill were caused by the estrogen component, scientists began experimenting to see whether the pill would still work if the amount of estrogen was reduced. It was found that the estrogen level could be reduced from about 100 micrograms to 50 or 30 micrograms and the pill would still work to prevent pregnancy. Most of the pills in use since 1969 have either 50 or 30 micrograms of estrogen. These do produce fewer cardiovascular side effects but the serious side effects are not completely eliminated. The lower-dose pills are also associated with a higher incidence of spotting (sporadic bleeding) than the high-dosage estrogen pill.

The 50 to 30 microgram estrogen pills do have one other disadvantage compared with the 100 microgram estrogen pills. If a woman forgets to take a 50 microgram estrogen pill, she is protected from pregnancy for only about 24 hours; if she forgets to take a 30 microgram pill, she is protected for about 12 hours. The higher-dose estrogen pills have the advantage of giving longer and more reliable protection from pregnancy in case a pill is forgotten.

In the hope of improving upon the safety of the oral contraceptive pill, much attention is now again being given to the progestin-only pill (minipill). If only the progestin is employed, will it be a safer form of contraception? The minipill has been used widely only since 1971. Because there is evidence which suggests that the progestin of the minipill is partly converted into estrogen by the body, it seems unlikely that all of the combined pill's serious problems can be avoided. It is known that the minipill can raise blood pressure, so at least one serious side effect is not completely eliminated.

The reason the minipill has not been used as extensively as the combined pill has to do both with the method of its administration and its efficacy in preventing unwanted pregnancies. Unlike the combined contraceptive pill which is taken for three weeks of every four, the minipill must be taken *every* day, and it is less effective in preventing pregnancy than the combined pill. The combined pill is about 20 times as effective as the minipill in preventing pregnancy. (The minipill has about the same effectiveness as the intrauterine device [IUD].) A significant disadvantage of the minipill is that missing even one day's dosage can destroy its effectiveness. Since the minipill must be taken every day, 365 days a year, this is a real problem. To overcome this, an injectable form of progestin is now available. The progestin is injected intramuscularly, and it is slowly absorbed into the body. This "injectable minipill" is available in some countries as Depo-Provera 150. An injection is necessary every 3 months.

To help you determine which type of contraceptive pill you may now be taking or may have taken in the past, the following table lists the name brands of the regular combined contraceptive pills, the low-dose combined pills, and the minipills.

THE COMBINED PILLS WHICH CONTAIN MORE THAN 50 MICROGRAMS OF ESTROGEN

Conovid	Enovid E	Ortho-Novum 1/80
Conovid E	Lyndiol 2.5	Ortho-Novum 2
Demulen*	Metrulen	Ortho-Novum 10
Enovid-5	Norinyl 1 + 80	Ovulen 1
Enovid-10	Norinyl 2	Ovulen 2

THE 30 MICROGRAM ESTROGEN COMBINED PILLS

Brevicon	Loestrin 20†	Ovamin 30
Brevinor	Lo/Ovral	Ovcon-35
Conova 30	Microgynon 30	Ovran 30
Demulen 30	Modicon	Ovranette
Eugynon 30	Neocon	Ovysemen
Loestrin 1/20†	Norimin	Restovas
Loestrin 1.5/30		

THE 50 MICROGRAM ESTROGEN COMBINED PILLS

Anovlar-21	Minilyn	Orlest 21
Con-Fer	Minovlar	Ortho-Novum 1/50
Demulen*	Minovlar ED	Ovcon-50
Demulen 50	Norinyl 1/28	Ovral
Eugynon 50	Norinyl 1	Ovran
Gynovlar 21	Norinyl 1 + 50	Ovulen 50
Microgynon 50	Norlestrin 1/50	Ovulen 1/50
Microgynon 50 ED	Norlestrin 2.5/50	Sequilan ED

THE MINIPILLS

Demovis	Micronor	Norgeston
Dianor	Micronovum	Noriday
Exluton	Microval	Noridei
Exlutena	Mikro-30	Norluten
Exlutona	Min-PE	Nor-Q.D.
Femulen	Neogest	Orgametil
Follistrel	Nordrogest	Orgametril
Microlut	Norfor	Ovrette
Micronett		

*In the United States Demulen has more than 50 micrograms of estrogen. In England Demulen has 50 micrograms of estrogen.
†Contains 20 micrograms of estrogen.

THE PILL RAISES BLOOD PRESSURE

All contraceptive pills can cause a rise in blood pressure, and the blood pressure tends to be higher the longer the pill is taken. The average rise in blood pressure is about 4.5 mg Hg systolic and 1.5 mm Hg diastolic. About 5 percent of women who take the pill for more than five years will develop true high blood pressure. That is, about 5 percent of women will develop a blood pressure of 140 mm Hg systolic or greater or 90 mm Hg diastolic or greater. The mechanism for this rise in blood pressure is not known. It is thought to be related to the estrogen component of the pill, but recent studies have demonstrated that the minipill (progestin only) can also cause the blood pressure to rise. Possibly this is because some of the progestin gets converted to estrogen by the body. When the pill is stopped, the blood pressure usually returns to normal levels within six months to one year. Occasionally the blood pressure never returns to normal levels. In this case, it is thought that the pill has brought out a woman's underlying tendency to have essential or primary hypertension.

You might think that an average rise of only 4.5 mm Hg systolic or 1.5 mm Hg diastolic is so small that it can be discounted. Can it? No one knows. It is known that a lower blood pressure is *always* better than a higher one. Statistics from life insurance companies have clearly proven that a small elevation of blood pressure over a period of time can significantly reduce life expectancy. How small is small? If your systolic pressure was 138 before the pill and 142 after the pill, you would receive an adverse rating from a life insurance company if you applied for insurance, because life insurance companies have data which prove that an individual whose blood pressure is 142 mm Hg systolic is a greater risk than one whose blood pressure is 138 mm Hg systolic. What if your systolic increases from 125 to 129? Is this significant? No one knows for sure, but it probably is. The best thinking is that there is some risk from this elevation, although the extent of the risk is difficult to quantitate. Do you want to take this risk?

Suppose the pill causes you to have true high blood pressure. Can you stay on the pill and take blood pressure medicine? If the blood pressure medicine fully corrects the rise in blood pressure produced by the pill, is it safe to take it? Most physicians would strongly advise you to stop the pill under this circumstance. The mechanism by which the pill produces high blood pressure is not known. When the pill raises your blood pressure, it has obviously significantly altered some aspect of your metabolism. Even if blood pressure medication reverses the high blood pressure effect of the pill, there is no assurance that the underlying altered metabolism has been corrected. Your body may now have two abnormalities instead of one. The first abnormality is produced by the pill, which raises your blood pressure. The second abnormality is produced by the medication introduced to bring your blood pressure back to normal. Is the pill worth this risk? Isn't it better to allow your metabolism to return to normal by simply stopping the pill?

THE PILL INCREASES THE RISK OF HEART ATTACK

At one time, a doctor rarely ever treated a woman for a heart attack until after she had gone through the menopause. Women just didn't have heart attacks at a young age. They didn't, that is, until they either started smoking cigarettes or starting taking oral contraceptive pills. Now, women who take the oral contraceptive pill are at least four times as prone to a heart attack as they were before starting the pill. If a woman both takes the pill and smokes cigarettes, this risk is multiplied by ten. The combination of the oral contraceptive pill and heavy cigarette smoking increases the risk of heart attack to about forty!

When medical scientists report that women who do not smoke increase their chance of heart attack four times when they take the contraceptive pill, this does not mean that the risk increases by four in every woman. This is the average risk experienced by all nonsmoking women between the ages of 15 and 44 who take the pill. Certain groups of women who take the pill are at greater risk of having a heart attack than others. You already know that women who are overweight, or who have a high cholesterol, or who have diabetes mellitus, or who have a family history of high blood pressure, early heart disease, or stroke are at greater risk. These are independent risk factors for heart attack. You also know that women who have high blood pressure are at greater risk, and you have probably already guessed that older women are at greater risk than younger women.

If you are in your teens or early twenties, do not smoke, did not have high blood pressure before you started the pill, and have not developed high blood pressure on the pill, *and* have none of the other risk factors listed above, you have very little reason to fear a heart attack. However, no woman who smokes should take the pill even if her blood pressure is normal at all times. No woman over 35 should take the pill. No woman over 30 should take the pill if she has any of the other risk factors. You should know that even in the most favorable circumstances, your risk of having a heart attack goes up the longer you take the pill.

If you do not smoke, have a normal blood pressure, and are under 30 years of age but do have one of the other risk factors, should you take the pill? Your risk of heart attack will go up once you start the pill, but it will not go up a lot. The risk does increase the longer you take the pill. Consequently, if you do decide to take this risk, you should limit the time that you will take the pill. More than about three to five years may be too risky.

THE PILL INCREASES THE RISK OF STROKE

The story for stroke is very much like the story for heart attacks. Strokes are very rare in premenopausal women. The risk of stroke increases about four times when a woman starts the pill, and it increases about forty times if she is a heavy cigarette smoker and also takes the pill. High blood pressure, high cholesterol, diabetes, obesity, and a family history of high blood pressure, early heart disease, or stroke are all independent risk factors for stroke, and women who take the pill and also have one of these risk factors are at greater risk than women who take the pill but have none of these risk factors. Older women are at more of a risk than younger women. For some reason, the risk of stroke goes up when a woman who suffers with migraine headaches takes the pill, and neurologists strongly recommend that women who have migraine headaches not take the pill.

The message seems clear. If you have high blood pressure, do not take the pill. If you develop high blood pressure while taking the pill, you should stop it. Even if you have a normal blood pressure, you should not take the pill if you smoke. If you are over the age of 30 and have any other risk factor, do not take the pill. Do not take the pill if you are over 35 years of age. If you are under 30 but have any of the other risk factors, you must recognize that you are at increased risk of stroke.

The risk of stroke goes up the longer you take the pill. This is very important and very serious information, because your risk of stroke is *not* entirely reversed when you stop the pill. All premenopausal women, whether they take the pill or not, are uniquely susceptible to a certain type of hemorrhage and stroke called *subarachnoid hemorrhage,* a rare but extremely serious condition. It is at least four times more common in women who take the pill, and the danger is even greater if other risk factors are present. Subarachnoid hemorrhage is much more likely to occur in women who take the pill and also smoke. Again, what is disturbing is the fact that the risk of this complication is not entirely eliminated once the pill is stopped.

Estrogens and progestins are members of a class of hormones called *steroids.* Steroids have profound effects upon the body. One thing they tend to do is alter the internal layers of arteries. The changes that they produce can make the arteries of the brain more susceptible to rupture. These are permanent changes and probably are more pronounced the longer the pill or other steroid is taken. This information should make every woman think very long and very hard before taking the pill. It should certainly convince any woman who smokes, or who has high blood pressure, or who has any of the other risk factors that the benefit of the pill is not worth this risk. It should also convince any woman that no matter how favorable her health is otherwise, she should limit the total length of time that she will use the pill as a method of contraception. How long? Based upon the available information, three to five years seems long enough.

THE PILL INCREASES THE RISK OF A BLOOD CLOT IN A VEIN

This section is added for the sake of thoroughness. In all the previous sections the particular complication of the pill was made more likely to occur if high blood pressure was also present. The presence of high blood pressure does not increase the chances of your forming a blood clot in a vein. However, this is a frequent complication of the pill, and you should be aware of it. Your risk of forming a clot in a vein increases about seven times when you take the pill. If you also smoke, this rises to about 21 times. Unlike the risk of heart attack and stroke, the risk does not go up the longer you take the pill. As soon as you start the pill, you experience this risk, and the risk stays about the same no matter how long you continue this form of contraception. Age, blood pressure, family history, and obesity all increase the likelihood of this complication from the pill. The added risk of developing a clot in a vein is eliminated when you stop the pill.

SHOULD *ANY* WOMAN TAKE THE PILL?

It seems clear that you should not take the pill if you have high blood pressure or if you develop high blood pressure while you are taking the pill. Since this is a book about high blood pressure, the chapter now could end. However, you are entitled to know the current thinking on behalf of the pill. An understanding of this topic is of critical importance to every woman of childbearing age.

Every woman who becomes pregnant runs the risk of dying from a complication of pregnancy or childbirth. To decide whether or not the pill is justified as a method of preventing pregnancy, the risk of a woman dying from a complication of the pill is compared with her risk of dying from either a complication of the pregnancy or a complication of childbirth. If the risk of dying from pregnancy or childbirth far exceeds the risk of dying from the pill, then it is thought by the medical profession that it is justified to expose a woman to the risk of the pill.

In certain countries the risk of dying from pregnancy or childbirth is very great. These are *developing nations* and include, for example, many nations of Africa and the Far East. In certain other countries the risk of dying from pregnancy or childbirth is not very great. This is true for the so-called *developed nations*. The United States, Canada, and the nations of Europe fall into this latter category. Fortunately, the improved nutrition and medical care available to women who live in the developed nations have greatly reduced the risks attendant to bearing a child. In Bangladesh almost 200 women out of every 100,000 can be expected to die during pregnancy or childbirth. When this is compared to the expected 10 to 20 deaths in this same population that will occur from the oral contraceptive pill, it may be reasonable to argue that it is justified to subject the women of Bangladesh to the risks of the pill. This argument can be made even stronger when it is pointed out that cultural factors make it impractical to gain widespread acceptance of alternative forms of contraception even though these are safer than the pill.

Can such an argument be made to justify exposing women who live in developed countries to the risks of the pill? Let's consider American women between the ages of 20 and 24. Their risk of dying during pregnancy or childbirth is about 5.8 women out of every 100,000. What is the risk of this same group of women dying from the oral contraceptive pill? It is 1.3 women out of every 100,000 as long as there are no smokers in the group. It goes up to 4.4 for the smokers. When 5.8 is compared to 1.3, it looks like a pretty good case can be made that the pill protects nonsmokers against death from pregnancy or childbirth. However, let's look at the risk of dying if some other form of contraception is used. This risk of dying is only 1.0 for every 100,000 women if the IUD is used, and it is only 0.3 when the diaphragm or condom is used backed up by medical abortion. If the purpose of contraception is to most effectively reduce the risk of dying from complications of pregnancy or childbirth, then the correct contraceptive method to choose is the one with the lowest risk, and that would be the diaphragm backed up by medical abortion.

You could conclude from this argument that there is no medical justification for women who live in America and the other developed nations to use the pill. The justification would have to be on the basis of convenience and effectiveness in preventing unwanted pregnancy. The older a woman gets, the weaker this justification is, for as a woman gets older, her risk of dying from a complication of the pill rises slightly more rapidly than the risk of dying from a complication of childbearing. If a woman smokes, it becomes very hard ever to justify the use of the pill, because by age 30 the risk of the pill equals the risk of childbearing, and by age 35 it is safer to be pregnant than it is to take the pill!

The decision whether or not to take the pill is indeed a difficult one, but it is not so difficult to make if you have high blood pressure. To return to the topic to which this book is dedicated: If you have high blood pressure, do not smoke. If you have high blood pressure, do not take the pill. If you have high blood pressure and also smoke, don't even think about taking the pill!

11

IF YOU TAKE THE FEMALE HORMONE ESTROGEN

Women who do not smoke or do not take the pill are seemingly protected against heart attacks and strokes until they go through the menopause. Once a woman goes through the menopause, her risk of suffering a heart attack or stroke increases about threefold. From that time on, the risk slowly rises as she grows older. At any age, the risk of heart attack and stroke is less for women than it is for men of the same age if all other risk factors are the same.

Why are women relatively protected from heart attacks and strokes? Medical scientists once thought that this was due to the female hormone, estrogen, since this hormone is unique to women. They even tried giving estrogen to men to see if it would protect them from heart attacks. They soon found it necessary to terminate this experiment, because the men who took the estrogen died at a faster rate than the men who did not take it. Then the data about the contraceptive pill started to come in, and it was learned that premenopausal women who take the pill have more strokes and heart attacks than premenopausal women who do not take the pill. The data strongly implicate the estrogen component of the pill as the agent which produces the adverse effects in the women of childbearing age.

The truth is that nobody understands why women of child-bearing age are protected against heart disease and stroke. It is logical that nature should have made this arrangement to ensure our survival; however, one cannot make a case that it is the female hormone estrogen which provides childbearing women with this biological protection. The extensive studies of the contraceptive pill clearly implicate the estrogen component as the cause of increased heart attacks and strokes in premenopausal women. In spite of this, the use of estrogen-containing medicines among women is extremely common. For example, at any one time, about one American woman out of every nine between the ages of 44 and 65 is taking an estrogen and about 70 percent of all American women between the ages of 44 and 65 years of age have used an estrogen. Is this a safe thing for this significant proportion of menopausal and postmenopausal women to do?

Since estrogens are so widely used, you might think that studies have been performed to decide this immensely important question. You would think that doctors know whether or not estrogen preparations given during or after menopause make women more susceptible to heart disease and stroke or less susceptible. Bad news. Very few studies have yet been performed, and there is much controversy among doctors about the relative merits and dangers of estrogens. Some doctors think that estrogens are the fountain of youth and should be taken forever by every woman who goes through menopause, whether the menopause is natural or produced by surgery. Other physicians believe there is no medical benefit to be obtained from estrogens beyond the relief they provide to lessen the uncomfortable symptoms associated with the menopause.

Some doctors argue that estrogens are justified because they help to prevent premature loss of calcium from bones, a process known as *osteoporosis*. Other doctors point out that this condition does not affect every woman who goes through menopause (in fact, it affects less than one woman in four), and that, to be effective, the estrogen must be started when a woman is quite young. Estrogens can help to protect bones from thinning but they work best if given *before* the problem begins. Obviously, it is very difficult to predict which woman will experience premature osteoporosis. Some experts recommend that estrogens are most helpful to women who undergo a premature menopause either because they undergo a surgical procedure which causes them to lose both ovaries at a young age, or because for some reason they just stop menstruating at an early age (for example, in the mid to late thirties).

Should a woman who goes through a natural menopause in her mid to late forties or early fifties be given estrogen replacement on the chance that she might be one who will experience premature thinning of the bones? This is a difficult question, and medical scientists do not have the answer. Many women may be able to protect themselves from this condition by remaining physically active, because it is known that regular physical activity helps to keep bones strong. If you and your doctor do decide that estrogen replacement therapy is desirable to protect your bones, you should know these facts: (1) For those who will benefit from estrogen replacement therapy, only a *low* dosage of the estrogen is necessary. There is no added advantage to taking a large dosage of the estrogen. For example, the equivalent of 0.625 mg of a conjugated estrogen preparation taken once per day is sufficient. (2) Unless you have had an operation which has resulted in the removal of your uterus (womb), the estrogen should be taken cyclically, which means the estrogen should be taken daily for three weeks, stopped for one week, and then started all over again. This partially imitates the normal menstrual cycle and has been shown to protect you at least somewhat from the increased risk of cancer of the uterus which is associated with replacement estrogen therapy.

It is now known that estrogen replacement therapy increases a woman's risk of developing cancer of the uterus by two- to eightfold. The risk increases the longer the estrogen is taken. The cyclic method of estrogen administration is thought to significantly protect against cancer of the uterus, and the addition of progestin to the cyclic program is thought to provide even greater protection. Many experts now recommend the following cyclic method of estrogen-progestin administration: Take an estrogen daily for 14 days. On day 15, add a progestin, so that both an estrogen and progestin are taken daily on days 15 through 21. Take no medication on days 22 through 28, and then start all over again. The estrogen dosage should be equivalent to about 0.625 mg of a conjugated estrogen preparation. The progestin dosage should be equivalent to about 10 mg of medroxyprogesterone. Present evidence suggests that the cyclic estrogen-progestin program is the safest program to follow if estrogen replacement therapy lasts longer than one year, because the addition of the progestin more closely imitates the normal menstrual cycle. During the fourth week, when no medication is taken, there is shedding of the cells which line the wall of the uterus, and this avoids the potential build-up of tissue that can result when only an estrogen is taken. Of course, if your uterus has been removed, it is unnecessary to take the progestin, and the estrogen can be taken every day instead of only 21 days out of every 28.

No doctor can argue that estrogens either increase or reduce the risk of heart attack and stroke. The studies haven't been done in sufficient numbers to find out. Furthermore it is possible that an estrogen has a different effect on a postmenopausal woman than it does on a premenopausal woman. (For obvious reasons, the studies of the contraceptive pill involved the premenopausal women.) Since it *is* known that estrogens raise blood pressure, and since an elevated blood pressure is never a good thing, it seems appropriate to advise you *not* to take an estrogen preparation if you have high blood pressure. It also seems appropriate to advise you to stop taking an estrogen preparation if you develop high blood pressure. This advice gives little comfort to women who are experiencing the discomforts of menopause. Does the symptomatic relief that is temporarily gained by taking an estrogen warrant the risk? It is not clear that this risk is justified for *any* woman. For the woman who has high blood pressure, present evidence suggests that this risk is too great.

If your doctor has prescribed estrogens for you, find out the reason why they were prescribed. Were you complaining of such persistent hot flashes and sweats that your doctor sat down with you and explained the potential risks of the medicine and the conflicting opinions about its safety, and then the two of you decided *together* that the benefit warranted the risk? Were you informed of the data which strongly suggest that long-term estrogen therapy increases the incidence of cancer of the uterus (womb)? Was it explained to you that estrogen may cause or aggravate fluid retention? Were you cautioned that your blood pressure might rise? If you were told that estrogen protects your bones from losing calcium, were you also told that this beneficial effect works best if you start the estrogen when still quite young and that osteoporosis affects less than one woman in four? What were you told of the possible relationship of estrogen to heart attack and stroke? Were you told that estrogens may increase your risk of experiencing a blood clot in a vein and that women who take estrogens are more likely to develop gallstones than those who don't take estrogens? Finally, were you advised to have "cyclic" therapy?

No medicine is free from side effects. You must be certain that any medication you take provides sufficient benefit to warrant the risk of its side effects. Estrogens are not the elixir of youth. They are medicines like any other, and you must apply the same criteria when deciding whether or not to take an estrogen that you would when deciding about any other medication that you introduce into your body.

Some people forget all the ingredients in the medicine they take. The following list gives the brand name of many of the estrogen preparations so that you can find out whether a pill you are taking contains estrogen.

Many estrogen preparations are also available as vaginal creams. The estrogen in these locally applied creams gets into the bloodstream, and the creams are probably no safer than the pills. Long-acting estrogen preparations are also available; these are given by injection. There is seldom justification for giving an injectable form of estrogen to relieve menopausal symptoms. If you are receiving such injections from your doctor, you should ask why this method was selected.

ESTROGEN PREPARATIONS BY BRAND NAME

Amnestrogen
Aquadiol
Aquagen

Cavomen-F
Climestrone
Conest
Conjugated estrogens
Controvlar
Cyclodiene
Cyclo-Progynova

Declimax
Diethylstilbestrol
Dimenformon
Distilbene
Dyloform

Edrol
Enavid
Equigyne
Estigen
Estinyl
Estivex
Estrace
Estracon
Estradurin
Estralate
Estraldine
Estratab
Estratest
Estrofem
Estrogena L
Estro-Med
Estromone
Estrosenor
Estrovagin
Estroval
Estrovis
Estrovite
Ethy II
Evex
Evtonyl

Farmacyrol
Femacoid
Femestral
Feminone
Femogen
Formatrix

Gynetone
Gynoestral
Gynolett

Harmogen
Hormofemin Compound
Hormonin

Lynoral

Mecrol
Mediatric
Menest
Menformon A
Menogen
Menolet Sublets
Menopax
Menophase
Menotrol
Menoval
Menrium
Mepilin
Metrulen
Milprem
Mixogen

Neo-Estrone
Novoconestrone

Oestradin
Oestraldin
Oestro-Feminal
Oestropax Mornings
Ogen
Ovestin

Pabestrol
Pentovis
PMP
Premarin
Prempak
Presomen
Primodos
Primogyn-C
Primogyn-M
Progynon-M
Progynova
Promarit

SK-Estrogens
Sodestran
Stilbol
Stilphostrol

Tace
Tag-39
Testaval
Test-Estrin
Theelin
Thelestrin
Transannon
Trimone
Tylesterone

Wynestron

Zeste

12

IF YOU ARE PREGNANT OR NURSING

HIGH BLOOD PRESSURE AND PREGNANCY

High blood pressure and pregnancy are not a happy combination. Women who already have high blood pressure when they begin their pregnancy or who develop high blood pressure once they become pregnant run a much greater risk of either losing their baby or of delivering a baby that is underweight. Blood pressure numbers that under other circumstances would be considered to be either normal or only mildly elevated constitute a very serious threat to a pregnancy.

Ideally, your blood pressure at the beginning of pregnancy should not be greater than 125/75. If it exceeds this figure, there is already some risk that the pregnancy will not be successful.

The higher the blood pressure rises above 125/75, the greater the risk. For example, should your blood pressure rise to 144/94—numbers which under other circumstances would not be considered cause for alarm—the risk of losing the baby is four times greater than it was when the blood pressure was 125/75.

True high blood pressure during pregnancy is *very* serious. This is not to say that you cannot have a very normal and very wonderful baby if you have high blood pressure. You can. It does mean that your pregnancy is more likely to end either in stillbirth or in delivery of a baby of low birth weight.

Unfortunately, treatment of your high blood pressure with medication will not improve the outcome of your pregnancy. Even though blood pressure medications may bring your blood pressure down to normal and keep it there at all times, your risk of either losing the baby or delivering an underweight baby remains the same.

If you take a blood pressure medication while you are pregnant, you should understand that you are treating only your blood pressure. You are not improving your chances of having a successful pregnancy. Moreover, since any medications taken during pregnancy carry some risk of harming the developing baby, you should be certain that it is truly essential that your blood pressure be treated with medication. *The safest and most effective medication to treat high blood pressure during pregnancy is REST*, even if this necessitates hospitalization. Blood pressure medications should be employed only when your blood pressure rises so high that it threatens your health.

IMPROVING THE OUTCOME OF YOUR PREGNANCY

Because you cannot expect to improve your chances of a successful pregnancy by treating your high blood pressure with medicine, it becomes extremely important that you take whatever steps you can to *correct any other health condition* which might adversely affect your pregnancy. If you smoke, you should stop immediately. If you are overweight, you should begin a weight loss program to bring your weight down to usually no more than 145 to 155 pounds *before* you become pregnant. (Once you *are* pregnant, you should not attempt to lose weight.) You should drink only small amounts of alcohol. You should avoid *all* medicines unless they are absolutely essential to maintain your health. You should eat well-balanced meals and take an appropriate multivitamin supplement. You should obtain adequate rest, even if this means staying in bed throughout a large part of your pregnancy.

It is normal for blood pressure to fall slightly during the first three months of pregnancy. Beginning with the fourth month, blood pressure normally begins to go up, and by the time you are close to delivery you can expect your blood pressure to rise about 10 mm Hg. The largest rise occurs after the sixth month, and for that reason it is very important that you see your doctor at increasingly closer intervals as your pregnancy progresses. If at any point in your pregnancy your blood pressure begins rapidly to rise or if during one of your regular checkups it is found that you are beginning to have a large amount of protein in your urine, your doctor will probably advise strict bed rest, even if this means putting you in the hospital. If you have a serious blood pressure problem, it is unlikely that your doctor will allow your pregnancy to reach full term. As soon as your pregnancy is far enough along to be certain that the baby is mature, which is about 38 weeks, your doctor will probably recommend that labor be induced or that you have a cesarian section.

Many women today have decided to delay having their family until they have had the opportunity to begin their careers. Consequently, many women are getting pregnant in their late twenties or early thirties. If you know you have high blood pressure, it is suggested that you do not delay your pregnancy too long. Your age is not a risk factor for pregnancy, but as you grow older, there is more likelihood of other conditions developing to complicate your already existing blood pressure condition. If you and your husband know that you want children, it is probably better for you to start your family earlier in your marriage than you might otherwise have planned.

WHAT YOU SHOULD KNOW ABOUT FLUID RETENTION

It is normal for women to retain fluid when they are pregnant. Puffy feet and ankles, puffy hands, and puffy eyelids are common and do not indicate that there is anything wrong. Fluid retention is not a cause for worry. It is an annoyance but *not* a health condition, and *you should not take a diuretic simply to get rid of fluid.* Diuretics are potent medicines, and like any other medication, a diuretic can harm your developing baby. No medicine should be taken during pregnancy unless it is truly required to correct a serious health condition of the mother. If you retain fluid, do not be concerned. If you wish to get rid of the fluid, limit the salt in your diet and lie down frequently. Lying down or sitting with your feet up helps the fluid get to your kidneys so that it can be excreted.

IF YOU DEVELOPED HIGH BLOOD PRESSURE WHEN YOU TOOK AN ORAL CONTRACEPTIVE PILL

Finally, some good news. If you developed high blood pressure when you took the pill, this does not mean that you will develop high blood pressure during pregnancy. There is no relationship between the blood pressure effect of the pill and the blood pressure effect of pregnancy.

IF YOU MUST TAKE HIGH BLOOD PRESSURE MEDICATION WHILE YOU ARE PREGNANT

In order to protect *your* health, your doctor may have to give you medication to control your blood pressure during your pregnancy. The available data suggest that women who take blood pressure pills have a slightly lower chance of having a successful pregnancy than women who do not take blood pressure medication. At first glance, this might seem to implicate the medication, but this is probably not correct. The correct interpretation is that women who require blood pressure medication also have the most serious blood pressure problems. The reason that women who take medication to treat blood pressure have more stillborns and more low-birth-weight babies is that these women also have the most advanced blood pressure problems. If blood pressure medicines are required, the increased risk to the baby is probably small. All the medications discussed in Chapter 7 can be used, but there are some that are best avoided. *Diuretics* should not be used alone, because they have not been shown to be very effective in controlling blood pressure elevation in pregnancy. They should be used only in conjunction with one of the other blood pressure medications. *Guanethidine* is best avoided because it can depress the baby's intestinal activity. *Reserpine* is best avoided because it can produce nasal stuffiness and a slow heart rate in the newborn. *Prazosin* and *minoxidal* are too new and there is not enough information to be certain of their safety; consequently, they probably should not be taken during pregnancy. *Methyldopa, clonidine, hydralazine,* and the *beta-blockers,* however, all may be relatively safe.

IN BRIEF

The presence of an elevated blood pressure before pregnancy or the development of high blood pressure during pregnancy is a serious threat to a successful pregnancy. High blood pressure medications do not improve the outcome of a pregnancy even when they successfully bring blood pressure down to normal and keep it there. You should take blood pressure medication only if blood pressure rises high enough to threaten your own health. The best way to ensure a good outcome of your pregnancy is to correct any other condition which can adversely affect pregnancy. If you have high blood pressure and become pregnant, or if you develop high blood pressure after you become pregnant, rest is essential. *Adequate rest* is the safest and most effective treatment of high blood pressure during pregnancy, and it is perfectly justified to be hospitalized if this is the only way complete rest can be assured. Fluid retention is not harmful to the developing baby and does not in any way affect pregnancy outcome. Consequently, you should not take diuretics simply to relieve the discomfort of fluid retention.

If blood pressure must be treated during pregnancy, a diuretic should be taken only in conjunction with one of the other classes of high blood pressure medicines. It should not be taken alone.

HIGH BLOOD PRESSURE MEDICINE AND NURSING

Little research has been performed to determine which of the high blood pressure medicines appears in breast milk in high enough concentrations to present a danger to the baby. As discussed in Chapter 7, almost every medicine that you take will enter your breast milk. Some medicines enter the breast milk freely, others in small amounts only. Because there is so little reliable information available, it seems best to advise you *not* to breastfeed your baby if you must take a blood pressure medication. Although there are certainly many desirable reasons to choose breastfeeding over bottle feeding, the advantages of breastfeeding probably do not outweigh the potential risks that blood pressure medications present to the baby.

Reserpine, guanethidine, propranolol, and diuretics are known to appear in breast milk. Although the concentrations are reported to be small, it seems unwise to expose your baby to even tiny amounts of any unnecessary chemical. No reliable information is available about the other blood pressure medicines.

It is unfortunate that material dealing with such an important topic should be so brief. Physicians and scientists simply haven't paid sufficient attention to this important subject. It is to be hoped that with women becoming increasingly interested in breastfeeding their babies, more research will be performed in the future. More complete information is needed not only about the effect that blood pressure medicines may have upon the nursing infant, but also about the potential effect that *any* medication taken by the mother may have on her baby.

13

IF YOU ARE A PARENT

Essential or primary hypertension runs in families. If you have essential hypertension, your child is at some risk of developing high blood pressure. Fortunately, there are ways that you can protect your child. Excessive salt consumption, obesity, and sedentary behavior are important contributors to the development of high blood pressure in children. All parents, whether they are victims of high blood pressure or not, should protect their child from foods which contain an excessive amount of salt. All parents should work hard to ensure that their child remains physically active and avoids excessive weight gain. It is especially important that parents who have high blood pressure take these steps. Preventive medicine is certainly the best medicine. If you can instill good diet and exercise habits early, you will not only significantly reduce the likelihood that your child will develop high blood pressure, but will also significantly reduce the possibility that your child will develop premature heart disease, stroke, or circulatory disease later in life.

WHAT YOUR PEDIATRICIAN OR FAMILY DOCTOR SHOULD DO

When your child reaches 3 years of age, it is time to start measuring blood pressure. From this time on, blood pressure should be checked at least once a year. A child's blood pressure is measured with the same type of blood pressure equipment that is used for adults. As in the case of adults, it is very important that the cuff be the correct size. It should cover two-thirds of the upper arm (between the elbow and the shoulder). A cuff that is smaller than this can give a falsely high blood pressure reading, and one that is larger can give a falsely low reading. Since children come in all sizes and shapes, it is important that the doctor have a variety of blood pressure cuffs from which to choose.

How will the doctor decide if the blood pressure is too high? This is not an easy question to answer, for it is normal for blood pressure to rise as a child grows older. A 6-year-old is con-

sidered to have an elevated blood pressure if the systolic pressure
is above 115 or the diastolic pressure is above 75. By age 9 the systolic pressure will have to be above 125 or the diastolic pressure
above 85 before the blood pressure is considered to be too high. By
the time a child reaches 12 years of age, the criteria employed to
define high blood pressure are the same as those used for an adult,
namely, a systolic pressure of 140 or greater or a diastolic pressure
of 90 or greater (see Chapter 4). Because the definition of high
blood pressure changes each year of a child's life up to age 12, your
child's blood pressure should be recorded on a specially designed
blood pressure graph called a *blood pressure grid.* The blood pressure grid allows the doctor to decide immediately when blood
pressure is too high at any age. Many but not all pediatricians and
general practitioners know about these grids and use them. Check
to make sure that your child's doctor is familiar with this helpful
device. Any doctor not presently using these grids can obtain them
from the High Blood Pressure Information Center, 120/80, Na-
tional Institutes of Health, Bethesda, Maryland 20014.

    If one of your children is discovered to have an elevated
blood pressure, the child should be given the three-part examination described in Chapter 5. If the child is less than 12 years old,
there is a high likelihood that after performing the medical history, the physical examination, and the basic set of laboratory
tests, the doctor will discover an underlying medical or surgical
condition which has caused the elevated blood pressure. If your
child is 12 or older, it is more likely that the examination will result in a diagnosis of essential or primary hypertension. Below the
age of 12, the most likely cause of high blood pressure is kidney
disease. Above this age, essential hypertension predominates, and
by age 20 the other causes of high blood pressure are relatively
rare.

    The medical and surgical conditions that can cause high
blood pressure in children are easily detected by the medical history, the physical examination, and the basic set of laboratory
tests. If the doctor gives your child a careful and thorough exam,
it is unlikely that an underlying kidney disease, hormonal imbal-
ance, or developmental abnormality will go unrecognized. Special
blood and urine tests and special X-rays are seldom necessary to
arrive at an accurate diagnosis.

    The medical and surgical conditions which can cause high
blood pressure were described in Chapters 6 and 9. In addition,
there are certain kidney diseases which can cause high blood pressure which are encountered mainly in children. A streptococcal infection, such as a streptococcal sore throat, tonsillitis, or skin infection, may occasionally lead to a kidney condition called

glomerulonephritis. This condition is easily diagnosed from the medical history and the routine examination of the urine. The majority of the children who develop glomerulonephritis recover completely, and their high blood pressure is only temporary.

Children are also susceptible to a condition called the *nephrotic syndrome.* The cause of this condition is not known. It is characterized by an excessive leakage of protein into the urine, a condition that is readily identifiable during routine examination, because one of the basic laboratory tests detects protein in the urine. It should be noted that usually the nephrotic syndrome is mild and does not cause high blood pressure. Only in the unusual advanced case is high blood pressure a problem.

Occasionally an infection or a developmental abnormality can cause the drainage tract from a kidney to become either partially or completely blocked. This causes back pressure on the kidney and produces a condition known as *hydronephrosis.* This is frequently detected during the physical examination because the enlarged kidney can be felt through the abdomen. The blood tests performed as part of the basic set of laboratory tests will also provide strong clues if this condition is the underlying cause of a child's high blood pressure.

If medication is required to treat your child's high blood pressure, the doctor will follow the same guidelines and use the same medications that were described in Chapter 7. The same blood pressure medications are used for everyone with high blood pressure, the same side effects occur, and the same precautions must be followed. You may think that it is complicated to decide the correct dosage of a child's medication because children vary so much in size and weight. Actually, the selection of medication dosage is quite simple. The dosage of any medication given to a child is based upon *weight.* There are standard formulas for each medication, and they allow the doctor to easily and accurately determine the correct dosage of any required medication. Under no circumstances should you assume that because you and your child are taking the same medicine, you can give your child your pills. Children require considerably less medication than adults. Remember that *the dosage of a child's medicine should always be based upon the child's weight and not upon the child's age.*

Some parents fear that a blood pressure medication may stunt their child's growth or sexual development. This is not true. None of the medications employed in the treatment of high blood pressure has been demonstrated to have such effects. As with adults, however, as few medications as possible should be used. In this regard, it is very important that proper attention be given to salt restriction, weight loss, and regular exercise.

WHAT PARENTS MUST DO

If one of your children is found to have high blood pressure, you must be certain that *all of your children are examined*. Even if the others are found to have normal blood pressures, you must be sure that they are reexamined at least once a year. The chance that high blood pressure may occur increases as a child grows older, and you must not develop a false sense of security because the blood pressure is now normal. Whether your child has high blood pressure or not, you must modify your family's diet so that foods served provide no more than about 5 grams of salt per day (see Chapter 8), and it is essential that you *teach* this diet to your entire household. If you can teach your children early in life to get along without using the salt shaker and to avoid foods which contain an excessive amount of salt, you may be able to prevent them from *ever* developing essential hypertension with all its attendant problems. Fortunately, public pressure has forced food manufacturers to stop adding salt to prepared baby foods. Unfortunately, many of the other foods which your child has learned to love so well and which are so abundantly available are very high in salt. As noted in Chapter 8, pizza, hot dogs, lunch meats, pickles and relish, ketchup, canned soups, canned vegetables, TV dinners, most baked pastry goods, many cereals, and most of the food served in the increasingly popular fast food restaurants all contain salt in excessive amounts. Your child gets a total of about 1.75 grams of salt from consuming one Big Mac, or one Burger King Whopper (close to 1 gram of salt) plus one small bag of french fries (0.1 grams of salt) plus one apple pie (0.4 grams of salt) plus one vanilla shake (0.25 grams of salt). This, of course, is before your child adds the extra salt provided in those attractive little packets (0.4 grams per packet).

Most of the foods thus far mentioned are not noticeably salty to the taste. Now think of all the snack foods and chips your child likes which are so wonderfully crunchy and so obviously salty! Clearly, you have your work cut out for you. You must carefully control the types of food you bring into the house so that your child doesn't learn from you to like those foods which are best avoided. You will have to be firm about snack and junk foods. They look appetizing when advertised on TV, and you have to resist the pressure your child will place upon you to buy them. If the adults in the household don't use the salt shaker, there is less chance that the children will learn this habit. You will have to carefully read the label of the canned and packaged foods that you buy to determine their salt content. True, fewer lunch meats, hot dogs, TV dinners, and fast foods may mean more work time in the kitchen. True, prepared, processed, and snack foods may be time-saving and convenient, but if they mean the early onset of heart disease, stroke, or circulatory disease in someone you love, are they worth it?

More than one-half of all children who develop high blood pressure are overweight. Correcting childhood obesity is very difficult, and it is also much more difficult for an adult to lose weight who was overweight as a child. You should make every effort to *prevent your child from ever becoming* overweight. One way to do this is to discourage snacking on candies, pastries, and ice cream. Since it is difficult to teach your child a diet and enforce the restriction of calories, a responsible weight loss program such as Weight Watchers or a program run by a nutritionist or dietician might provide helpful motivation. Another way to protect your child against obesity is to encourage regular participation in vigorous dynamic exercise (see Chapter 14). Overweight children generally are sedentary, and the lack of regular exercise is a significant contributor to their weight problem. *It is essential that a regular program of dynamic exercise be a part of the weight loss program.* Swimming, bicycling, and sports that require a lot of running are effective. Sports that require a good deal of arm motion, such as tennis, are less so.

You should not smoke cigarettes. It is unrealistic for you to expect your child to overcome the lure of the cigarette ads and the pressure of friends if you are a cigarette smoker.

You should not allow your child to use a salt substitute. If you choose to use a salt substitute (see Chapter 8), be certain to keep it well out of the reach of young children. The kidneys of even the healthiest youngster may not be able to handle the large amounts of potassium that a salt substitute contains.

GOOD HEALTH HABITS LAST A LIFETIME

Essential hypertension probably begins early in life. Medical scientists are only now beginning to study extensively the problem of high blood pressure in infants and youths. Each day brings new and convincing evidence that the changes which lead to heart disease, stroke, and circulatory disease start very early. It is now known that the fat deposits which lead to atherosclerosis may start as early as 3 to 5 years of age. High blood pressure is a potent contributor to the early development of atherosclerosis, and it is very likely that the level of blood pressure achieved as a child strongly influences the level of blood pressure in adult life. By encouraging your child to eat a diet that is low in salt and animal fats, to exercise regularly, and to avoid the cigarette habit, you will have done much to ensure lasting good health.

14

THE SAFE WAY TO EXERCISE IF YOU HAVE HIGH BLOOD PRESSURE

If you are a very active person and discover that you have high blood pressure, should you slow down? If you have led a fairly lazy life but wish to reform and start an exercise program, can you safely do so if you have high blood pressure? Are there certain kinds of physical activity that you should avoid if you have high blood pressure? Are there certain kinds of physical activity that may prove beneficial to your health? Can participation in the right kind of exercise program actually lead to a permanent lowering of blood pressure? If you are taking blood pressure medication, is it safe to exercise?

These are important questions, and the answers to these and other questions about the relationship between physical activity and high blood pressure are difficult to find. Your doctor may not be able to give you completely accurate advice. Most physicians do not know a great deal about exercise. Medical teaching emphasizes the recognition and treatment of disease, and the practicing physician has relatively little exposure to the topic of exercise. Unless your physician has a special interest in this subject or has received advanced training in cardiology, you may be cautioned to limit your physical activity more than is really necessary. You may not be informed that certain kinds of physical activity may prove beneficial to your health and that other kinds are best avoided. You may not be given sufficient warning about certain blood pressure medications.

In this chapter you will learn that it is generally safe and desirable for you to remain physically active if you have high blood pressure. You will learn that not only can you safely undertake a program of physical exercise if you have been mainly sedentary, but that the right kind of exercise program is probably beneficial to you and may even lead to a permanent lowering of your blood pressure.

THE TWO TYPES OF EXERCISE

There are two types of exercise. One type, *isometric exercise*, almost always causes a rise in blood pressure during its performance. The other type of exercise, *dynamic exercise*, only causes the blood pressure to rise when it is performed vigorously. *Individuals who have high blood pressure can almost always safely engage in some level of dynamic exercise.* Dynamic exercise leads to increase cardiovascular fitness, and participation in a regular program of dynamic exercise is to be encouraged. Isometric exercise leads to increased muscle strength and bulk, but it does not lead to increased cardiovascular fitness. All forms of vigorous physical activity produce a rise in blood pressure, but the rise in blood pressure produced by isometric exercise is generally greater than that produced by dynamic exercise. If you have high blood pressure, you should be encouraged to begin or to continue a program of regular dynamic exercise, but you should avoid strenuous isometric activities.

Isometric Exercise

Weight lifting is a classic example of an isometric exercise. Physical activities which require you to lift heavy objects or to strain or to pull against a resistance are isometric activities. This type of physical activity is characterized by a prolonged fixed contraction of a group of muscles. When you strain to hold the wheel of your car steady on a busy road, you are performing isometric exercise with the muscles of your hands and arms. When you shovel snow or hold a heavy bundle with your arms, you are performing an isometric exercise. When you press down on the brakes of your car and hold the brake down firmly, you are performing an isometric exercise with your leg muscles. The regular performance of isometric exercises produces an increase in the size and the strength of the muscles which are exercised.

Although isometric exercises improve muscle strength and bulk, they do not lead to an improvement in cardiovascular fitness. That is, they do not improve endurance. During the time that a group of muscles is held in fixed contraction, there is a rise in blood pressure. This can be dangerous if you have high blood pressure or heart disease, and the limited benefit you derive from isometric exercise does not justify the risk. Unless your job requires you to strengthen a specific group of muscles or you wish to play a sport that requires you to develop unusual muscle strength, you should generally avoid strenuous isometric exercise and those strenuous physical activities which are mainly isometric.

Many activities of daily life require you to perform some degree of isometric exercise. Most often, these are activities that employ the muscles of the arms and hands, such as shoveling, carrying bundles, squeezing, pressing, and pulling. Straining to have a bowel movement is also an isometric activity. Although it is not possible to avoid these activities completely, it is possible to modify them so there is only a small rise in your blood pressure during their performance. If you have to shovel, take only a little dirt or snow onto the shovel at a time. If you must carry bundles, keep them light and make more trips. Try to avoid vigorously straining to press, push, or pull an object. Get help with that stuck window. Don't volunteer to help push your neighbor's car or to move a heavy object. Leave this to those who have normal blood pressures and healthy hearts. If constipation is a problem, increase the amount of bran and fiber in your diet and use stool softeners and perhaps a mild laxative.

If you have high blood pressure, you should *not* employ isometric exercise as the major way to stay in shape or as your major form of recreational exercise. Lifting light weights and working out against a light resistance may be fine. This will keep your muscles toned up and may improve your appearance. However, you should not try to be a body builder. Many health spas, gyms, and exercise clubs now promote the use of weight machines which allow you to exercise many different groups of muscles. You should understand that the benefit of this type of exercise to your overall health is not great, and that if these types of resistance exercises are performed strenuously, your blood pressure will rise significantly while you are performing them. It requires only very light weights to firm up muscles and improve their tone. There is little health benefit to be derived from exercises which only build bigger muscles. They are not worth the risk. Cardiovascular fitness is improved by engaging in exercises that produce a sustained increase in the rate of your heartbeat. Such exercises are called dynamic exercises, and this is the type of physical activity you should use both for staying in shape and for recreation.

Dynamic Exercise

Walking, jogging, running, and swimming are classic examples of dynamic exercise. Muscles are moved naturally and rhythmically. They are never held in fixed contraction. As soon as the muscles contract, they immediately relax. If added weight or resistance is present, it is never enough to prevent the natural and even flow of muscular activity. Most of the physical activity which you perform with your legs is dynamic exercise. When you walk, you are performing dynamic exercise. When you walk while carrying a bundle, you are performing dynamic exercise with your legs and isometric exercise with your arms. When you swim you are performing dynamic exercise with both your arms and your legs. When you bicycle on a level surface and only lightly hold onto the handles with your hands and arms, you are performing dynamic exercise with your legs. When you bicycle up a hill and hold the handles with a firm grip and tensed arm muscles, you are adding isometric exercise with your hands and arms.

Almost everyone can safely engage in some level of dynamic exercise. The vigor of dynamic exercise is measured not by how much weight you lift but by how rapidly your heart beats. Mild dynamic exercise such as slow walking or bicycle riding usually is associated with only a small rise in the pulse rate. Although blood pressure may rise when you perform dynamic exercise, it will rise in proportion to the speed of your heartbeat. If you perform dynamic exercise so that there is only a slight rise in your pulse rate, your blood pressure may not rise at all. This is in sharp distinction to isometric exercise. Your pulse rate may not increase at all while you are lifting a heavy weight, but your blood pressure may rise to very high levels.

There are many health benefits to dynamic exercise. Participation in a regular program of dynamic exercise can lead to increased cardiovascular fitness (increased endurance), but it will not lead to an increase in either muscle size or muscle strength. Weight lifters gain weight when they train, joggers do not. The regular participation in dynamic exercise is more likely to lead to a weight loss than a weight gain. Many women are hesitant to undertake a jogging program because they believe it will lead to an increase in the size of their legs. This is not true. Jogging will lead to increased endurance but not increased muscle size. In fact, the combined effect of weight loss and improved muscle tone will most likely decrease the size of the buttocks, thighs, and calves. A program of dynamic exercise often produces a permanent lowering of blood pressure, and this is especially true if the blood pressure elevation is only mild to begin with. Many recreational activities (for example, tennis) require dynamic exercise. A regular program of dynamic exercise leads to improved endurance and should therefore lead to improved performance.

If you have been regularly participating in a sport or occupational activity which involves mainly dynamic physical activity and discover that you have high blood pressure, there is probably little reason for you to make any changes in your exercise program. In fact, it is most likely to your benefit to continue the activity. If you have been mainly sedentary and discover that you have high blood pressure, it will probably be to your benefit to start a program of regular dynamic exercise. It is true that vigorous dynamic exercise is associated with a rise in blood pressure during the time that you are exercising. In fact, if systolic blood pressure (top number) doesn't go up during vigorous dynamic exercise, this usually means that serious heart disease exists. Both normal individuals as well as those who have high blood pressure must experience some rise in the systolic blood pressure during the time that they are exercising. In the absence of heart disease, this is not dangerous. You will learn below that this rise in systolic blood pressure is a normal and essential response to dynamic exercise, and that it is not possible for you to safely engage in vigorous dynamic exercise unless your blood pressure does go up during this time. (Unless you have heart disease, diastolic pressure does not rise during dynamic exercises. It stays the same or falls slightly.)

Your doctor is probably correct in instructing you to stop shoveling snow and to stop lifting heavy objects once you are detected to have high blood pressure. Your doctor may not be correct in advising you to give up jogging, running, swimming, tennis, and other sports which involve mainly the rhythmic movement of your arms and legs without added resistance or added weight. In most instances, you should be encouraged to continue these activities if you perform them regularly, or to undertake such activities if you have been mainly sedentary. If there is any doubt about the safety of dynamic exercise, you can be given an exercise stress test. This test will determine with reasonable assurance the level of dynamic exercise which you can safely undertake. The vigor of dynamic exercise is measured by the pulse rate, and the rise in blood pressure is related to the rise in pulse rate. If you are properly tested, your doctor will be able to tell you how high your blood pressure rises at any given pulse rate. This will allow you to regulate the intensity of your exercise so that you keep your blood pressure within a safe range.

Why Blood Pressure Rises When You Engage in Vigorous Dynamic Exercise

During the time that you walk briskly, or jog, or run, your blood pressure will rise. Why is this a normal and necessary response? The muscles of your legs are rapidly expanding and contracting and these working muscles require a lot of food and oxygen to maintain their activity. In order to get more food and oxygen to the leg muscles, more blood must flow to them. The more vigorously the muscles work, the more blood they demand. During vigorous dynamic leg exercise, the flow of blood to the legs may increase as much as fifteen times what it is when the legs are at rest. In order to bring this extra blood to the leg muscles and protect the circulation of the brain, it is essential that blood pressure rise.

This is what happens: During dynamic leg exercise, the vigorously working muscles of the legs release chemicals which make the arteries bringing blood to these muscles dilate widely. It is like a dam which is suddenly opened—the water comes rushing through where once it flowed slowly. When the arteries to the working muscles are widely dilated, the blood rushes to them and the blood pressure in the legs suddenly drops to a low level. Blood is diverted away from the arms, abdomen, and the rest of the body and into the legs. Unless adjustments are immediately made in the rest of the circulation, this diversion of blood into the legs might prove dangerous. A rise in blood pressure in the rest of the body will have to occur to compensate for the drop in blood pressure in the legs; otherwise the brain will be deprived of blood, and this may lead to a loss of consciousness (faint).

As soon as the body senses that a large amount of blood has suddenly been diverted to the legs, the nervous system sends out the message, "Raise the blood pressure," to the arteries that take blood to the arms and to the organs in the abdomen. These arteries immediately constrict. This has two effects: (1) less blood flows to the arms and to the abdomen, and (2) blood pressure in the rest of the body goes up. At the same time that this is happening, the heart beats more rapidly. The working leg muscles require a continuous renewal of their supply of food and oxygen, and the blood must rapidly recirculate to remove the waste products produced by the working muscles and bring them the necessary food and oxygen. To keep the blood circulating rapidly, the heart has to beat more rapidly. The combined effect of the constriction of the arteries to the arms and abdomen and the increase in the pulse rate ensures that the blood pressure stays high enough to deliver sufficient blood to the brain at all times.

As exercise becomes increasingly vigorous, the muscles of the legs demand an even greater flow of blood. At first, the muscles are able to achieve an increase in the flow of blood by further dilating the blood vessels. This further lowers the resistance to flow, and blood rushes through. Eventually, a time comes when the blood vessels can become no wider, and this means that resistance can be reduced no further. Now there is only one way that the flow of liquid through the arteries can be increased: the heart must push on the blood more forcefully, causing the blood pressure to rise.

Thus, there are two reasons that your blood pressure goes up when you engage in vigorous leg activity. At first the rise in blood pressure is created by the compensatory constriction of the arteries in your arms and abdomen in response to the fall in blood pressure which occurs in your legs. The second rise in blood pressure results when the blood pressure in your legs can fall no further. To pump still more blood into your legs, your heart must now not only beat still more rapidly, but it must also push on the blood stream with greater force. This means, of course, that blood pressure must rise still further.

You do not have to be concerned that your blood pressure will continue to rise higher and higher the longer or more vigorously you exercise. Your body has a built-in mechanism to protect you. There is a limit to how fast your heart can beat, and this serves to limit how high your blood pressure can rise. Unfortunately, it also sets a limit on your endurance. As one gets older, there is a natural decrease in the maximum heart rate that can be achieved. Someone who is 30 years old may be able to achieve maximum heart rate of about 190 beats per minute. Someone who is 50 years old will be unable to raise the pulse rate much above 170 beats per minute. Because of this, there is a natural decline in the total amount of physical exercise that can be accomplished, and this is why older individuals have less endurance than younger individuals.

If you perform isometric exercise at the same time that you perform dynamic exercise, your blood pressure will rise more than when you perform only dynamic exercise. Let's see how this happens. Suppose you are walking very briskly while carrying a heavy package. While the muscles of your legs are rhythmically contracting and relaxing (dynamic), your arm muscles are held in fixed contraction (isometric). You know that in response to the increased demand for blood by your leg muscles, the arteries in your arms and abdomen contract, blood is diverted to the legs, and blood pressure goes up. When you hold muscles in fixed contraction, it is more work for the heart to pump blood through the arteries to these muscles, and the heart must beat even more forcefully to overcome this increased resistance to blood flow. Now the heart has to overcome not only the increased resistance to blood flow which results from the message to the arteries of the arms and abdomen, but also the added resistance to blood flow produced by the contracted arm muscles. Since the heart must beat still more forcefully, there is a further rise in blood pressure. Thus, isometric exercise causes a large increase in blood pressure because it is more work for the heart to pump blood through muscles which are held in fixed contraction. If you carry the weight of the package on your back by using a back pack, you will not experience as much of a rise in blood pressure.

Any activity which does not permit the muscles to rapidly contract and relax can elevate the blood pressure. For example, gripping the handles of a bicycle so tightly that the hand and arm muscles are quite tense will cause a bicyclist's blood pressure to rise more than when the arms and hands are held relaxed. You can see that when you perform dynamic exercise, you should use a natural and easy style and keep your muscles as relaxed as possible.

Isometric exercise raises blood pressure in relation to the amount of muscles that are held in the contracted state. The more muscles that are held in fixed contraction, the larger the rise in blood pressure. By rearranging a task, you can often avoid the rise in blood pressure which would otherwise occur. For example, carrying a heavy bag of groceries even a short distance may cause a large rise in blood pressure during the time that you are carrying it. If you carry only one or two items at a time, you will have to make many more trips but your blood pressure probably will not rise at all. Even though unloading the bag of groceries this way requires walking a longer distance, the extra walking probably will not significantly raise your blood pressure. It is not only always safer for you to perform dynamic exercise, but you will be able to safely accomplish *more* exercise if you concentrate on dynamic activities and avoid isometric activities.

You have seen that the more vigorously you perform dynamic leg exercise, the more blood is shunted away from the arms and abdomen and into the legs. Now you understand why you are always warned not to exercise vigorously until at least two hours after a large meal. When you eat a full meal (as opposed to a snack), the organs of digestion within the abdomen require a great deal of blood. However, if vigorously working muscles are diverting the blood away from the abdomen, this interferes with the digestive process and may cause painful stomach cramps.

EXERCISE STRESS TESTING AND MEASURING YOUR PULSE RATE

By performing an *exercise stress test,* your doctor will be able to tell you approximately what pulse rate produces what degree of blood pressure elevation. You can then count your pulse while you are exercising and in this way have reasonable assurance that you are staying within a safe blood pressure range.

If you are an active person and regularly participate in an occupation or a sports activity which involves mainly dynamic activity, there is little reason for you to stop or modify your activity if you are discovered to have high blood pressure. Unless you wish to considerably increase the vigor of your activity or unless you have easy shortness of breath, chest discomfort, or other symptoms which might indicate that you have underlying heart disease, there is little reason for you to undergo an exercise stress test. If you have not been very physically active but are under 35 years of age, do not smoke, and have only mild elevation of blood pressure, it is probably safe for you to begin a program of dynamic exercise without a stress test.

If you have a significant blood pressure elevation (above 110 mm Hg diastolic), if you are over 35 years of age, or if you have been a heavy cigarette smoker, you should consider having an exercise stress test before you begin a *new* program of dynamic exercise. This will accomplish two things: (1) you may find out if you have any underlying heart disease, and (2) you will find out how much your blood pressure rises as your pulse rate increases. This will allow you safely to regulate your level of exercise by counting your pulse, using a method that will be described later. If you have no underlying heart disease, it is safe for you to allow your systolic pressure to rise to about 200 to 250 mm Hg for about 20 minutes.

The stress test should be performed on either a special exercise bicycle, called *a bicycle ergometer*, or a treadmill. The exercise bicycle must have special adjustments so that the examining physician knows exactly how much work you are doing when you pedal at a steady rate of 50 revolutions per minute. The treadmill must have controls which allow both the speed and the incline of the treadmill to be adjusted. This allows the physician to test your ability to walk up a hill. The treadmill track should be wide enough and long enough for you to exercise with your usual comfortable, natural stride.

Before the test is performed, your doctor should give you a thorough physical examination, measure your blood pressure, and obtain a full electrocardiogram. Then a series of small adhesive patches should be applied to your chest so that the electrocardiogram can be observed *at the time that you are exercising.* It is essential that the physician performing the test have what is called a *heart monitor.* This looks like a TV screen, and it displays a continuous picture of your heart action while you are exercising. At one time, before more accurate equipment was available, stress tests were performed by taking a cardiogram, then having the individual exercise strenuously (usually by running up and down a platform of steps), and then taking another cardiogram immediately upon completion of the exercise activity. *This is unsatisfactory.* The electrocardiogram must be observed all the time that you are exercising as well as when you are through exercising. Furthermore, your blood pressure and pulse rate must be measured at frequent intervals while you are performing the exercise test (at least every three minutes). Once the exercise test is completed, it is necessary to continue to monitor your cardiogram, pulse, and blood pressure for about ten more minutes. This is called the *cooldown period,* and it is just as important to know what happens to your cardiovascular system during this period as it is to know what happens while you are actively exercising.

The exercise stress test is performed by gradually increasing either the work of bicycling or the speed and incline of the treadmill. Each level of exercise, called a *stage* of the exercise test, usually lasts from three to six minutes. Shorter intervals of exercise should not be used, because it takes between three to six minutes for the blood pressure to stabilize at any given pulse rate. At the end of each stage of exercise, a permanent tracing of the electrocardiogram should be obtained and your blood pressure should be recorded. The electrocardiogram tracing will give an accurate measure of how fast your heart is beating, whether the heart is under any strain, and whether there is any irregularity of the rhythm. If the test does not cause you to become too fatigued or to experience too much shortness of breath or to feel any chest discomfort, you should continue exercising until you reach what is called your *age-predicted maximum heart rate*. During the times that you are exercising, it is to be expected that your systolic blood pressure (top number) will rise and that the diastolic pressure will stay the same or fall slightly. If the systolic blood pressure falls, the test should be stopped immediately, for this usually means that heart disease exists.

To prepare yourself for an exercise stress test, you should have nothing to eat for at least two hours before the test is scheduled, and it is best to eat only a light meal at that. If you smoke (and it's best if you don't), do not smoke for at least two hours before the test. You should wear comfortable clothes and good pair of walking or exercise shoes. If you are taking any medications, you should take them as you usually do. Since you are taking the exercise stress test to determine the safe level at which you can exercise, it is important that you know what effect your medication will have upon your ability to exercise, particularly if you are taking any medication to treat high blood pressure.

As you will learn later in this chapter, it may be dangerous to engage in vigorous dynamic exercise if you are taking certain blood pressure medicines. An exercise stress test is an excellent way to test the safety of these medicines. You must be certain to tell the examining physician all the medicines that you take. Once the test is completed, you should plan to sit quietly for a while in the physician's office in order to cool off completely, and you should not take a hot shower for at least one hour after the test. Heat is potentially dangerous to those who exercise vigorously.

Once the exercise test is completed, you should ask the examining physician the following questions:

1. What is my age-predicted maximum heart rate?
2. What was my blood pressure before I started the stress test?
3. What heart rate did I achieve during the stress test?

    4. How high did my blood pressure rise during the stress test?

    5. What was my blood pressure at the end of the cool-down period?

    6. Did the test reveal any evidence of heart disease?

    7. Did the test reveal any disturbance of my heart rhythm?

    8. What is the safe level to which I can raise my heart rate for twenty minutes while I am exercising?

    If the test reveals any evidence of underlying heart disease, then you should ask the doctor to *specifically prescribe* an exercise program for you or to refer you to a facility which can offer you a *supervised exercise program.* The exercise recommendations in this chapter are intended for individuals who have high blood pressure but who have no evidence of underlying heart disease.

PULSE RATE AND PHYSICAL FITNESS

Many books about exercise are now available, and many commercial weight loss programs and health clubs offer regimens and advice to help you exercise. Usually, these books and programs teach you a method of exercise which involves counting your pulse. To a certain extent this is correct. You should, however, understand one thing: the extent to which your pulse rate rises when you exercise is one measure of the level of your physical fitness, *but it is not in any way an indicator of whether or not you have underlying heart disease.*

    Consider two individuals of the same age. One exercises regularly by mild jogging and the other does not exercise at all. Both are instructed to perform the same amount of exercise at the same intensity; for example, both are told to walk for ten minutes at three miles per hour. At the end of this activity, each counts the pulse rate. The individual who has been exercising regularly will have a lower pulse rate at the end of this activity than the one who has been mainly sedentary. All you learn from this is that the individual with the lower pulse rate is probably more physically fit for this particular walking activity (that is, has more endurance) than the individual who has the higher pulse rate. *You have not obtained any information to help you decide whether or not either individual has any degree of underlying heart disease.*

    The individual with the higher pulse rate may have a perfectly normal heart and just be out of shape. The individual with the lower pulse rate may be more physically fit for the walking activity but in fact have significant underlying heart disease. You have *not* learned, for example, that the individual with the lower pulse rate can safely start a running program, nor have you learned that the individual with the higher pulse rate cannot safely start a running program. Counting the pulse is *not* an exercise stress test. You should know this because many books and commercial exercise and weight loss programs lead you to believe that when they test you this way they are giving you a form of exercise stress test. This is not true, and you are not necessarily protected from the dangers of excessive physical activity simply because you achieve a lower pulse rate than someone else.

THE MEANING OF PHYSICAL FITNESS

What does improved physical fitness really mean? It means that you can perform a given amount of exercise with improved efficiency. Because you can perform the amount of exercise more efficiently, you can do more of it. Increased physical fitness means that you have increased your level of endurance. For example, if before you begin an exercise program you are fatigued after walking one mile briskly, then after you improve your level of physical fitness you may be able to walk three or more miles before experiencing the same feeling of fatigue. Increasing your physical fitness means that you have given your engine a good "tune-up." You get more mileage from the same amount of "gas." In this case, the gas is the oxygen and food that your muscles require. Just as an engine runs more smoothly when it is well tuned, so does your cardiovascular system.

One indicator of an improved cardiovascular performance level is the pulse rate. If before you begin a program of physical fitness your pulse rate reaches, say, 140 beats per minute after you walk one mile briskly, then after you have achieved an improved level of fitness your pulse rate may rise to only 120 beats per minute after the same amount of exertion. You can use your pulse rate as an indicator that you are improving your level of physical fitness, but remember that you cannot assume anything from your pulse rate about underlying heart disease. It may be that as you improve your level of physical fitness, you improve the health of your heart. There is information which suggests that this is so. Some medical studies seem to indicate that physically fit individuals have lower rates of death from heart attacks than unfit individuals. The thing to remember, however, is that physical fitness is relative. *You can have underlying heart disease and still improve your level of physical fitness.* You may still have the same amount of heart disease once you are more fit, but you will have trained your cardiovascular system to perform a given amount of exercise more efficiently. Even though the condition of your heart is not changed, your heart will have to perform *less* work to perform the activity once your level of fitness improves. This, of course, is very desirable, for you will then be able to safely engage in more physical activity.

When you improve your level of physical fitness, then, you protect your heart because your heart has to do less work to accomplish the same amount of exercise. Improved cardiovascular fitness results mainly from the improved ability of your muscles to utilize their food and oxygen supply. A program of regular dynamic exercise trains your muscles to get by with less oxygen and less food and still do the *same* amount of work. Since the muscles demand less food and oxygen, they also demand less blood. This means that your heart does not have to beat as forcefully or as rapidly to supply the working muscles. There may be some direct improvement in heart function as well, and there may even be an improvement in the flow of blood through the coronary arteries that directly supply the heart. However, it is important for you to understand the major beneficial effect of a program of regular dynamic exercise is improved muscle metabolism. This means that even individuals who have damaged hearts can improve their endurance, for even if the function of their heart cannot be improved, the increased efficiency of their muscles will permit the heart to perform more work.

HOW TO IMPROVE YOUR LEVEL OF PHYSICAL FITNESS

You improve your level of physical fitness by engaging in a regular program of dynamic exercise. The aim of your exercise program is to allow you to get "more miles per gallon." As you become more fit, you will be able to perform more exercise for a given amount of oxygen. Improved cardiovascular performance is what is desired, and not simply improved muscle strength. Remember that exercises that only increase the size and the strength of your muscles (isometric exercises) do not tune up your cardiovascular system. To tune up your cardiovascular system you must regularly participate in a program of exercises which speed up your pulse rate, and only dynamic exercises do this.

If you have high blood pressure and wish to improve your level of physical fitness, these are the important questions that you must ask:

1. What kind of dynamic exercise activities should I perform?
2. How should I perform these activities?
3. How high should my pulse rate go?
4. How long should I exercise at the desired pulse rate?
5. How many times per week should I exercise?
6. How can I tell if I am making any progress?

7. Once I am physically fit, what do I have to do to maintain this improved state of health?

8. If I improve my endurance by regularly performing one type of physical activity, can I assume that it is safe for me to perform other types of physical activity?

9. What precautions are necessary if I take blood pressure medications?

In the discussion that follows it is assumed that you either are under 35 years of age, do not smoke, and have only mild elevation of your blood pressure, or it is assumed that you are already exercising with some regularity or have undergone an exercise stress test and have been told that the test did not reveal evidence of underlying heart disease. Although the same basic principles are employed to improve physical fitness where there is underlying heart disease, such individuals need close medical supervision. Increased physical fitness is achieved by gradually increasing the level of exertion, and individuals with underlying heart disease should have their exercise stress test repeated at each stage of their program. This periodic checking is not necessary if you have no evidence of underlying heart disease, unless you wish to consider undertaking a very strenuous level of exercise.

1. The Recommended Kinds of Dynamic Exercise Activity

A *walking–jogging–running* program is the safest form of exercise for individuals who have high blood pressure. You will remember that blood pressure rises less when muscles are used rhythmically and naturally. Walking, jogging, and running are the most natural forms of exercise activity, and they are excellent endurance exercises. Pulse counting is necessary to monitor your program, and pulse counting is easier to do with this type of activity than any other. Walking, jogging, and running require no instruction and no special equipment. It can be performed in almost all weather conditions, and you are not dependent on a partner for your exercise. Also it does not require a great amount of time. The whole idea is to perform dynamic activity in the way that is most natural for you. If you have been mainly sedentary, you should not attempt any other exercise activity until you have participated in a walking–jogging–running program for about three months.

Bicycling is a good dynamic exercise activity, but it is not recommended as your initial exercise activity if you have been mainly sedentary. In the first place, stationary bicycling indoors is very boring, and few individuals stick with such a program very long. Second, most individuals do not live in a location where either automobiles or climate allow regular participation in a vigorous program of outdoor bicycling. It is also more difficult to count your pulse when bicycling. Finally, you should remember that when you bicycle vigorously, you have a tendency to grip the handles firmly and tense your arm muscles. This is isometric activity, and it can cause a rise in blood pressure. Individuals with more than a mild elevation of blood pressure and those who are over the age of about 55 should not employ bicycle riding as a serious exercise activity until they have first devoted a few months to a walking–jogging–running program.

Swimming is an excellent dynamic exercise activity, but it is difficult to start swimming at a low level of physical exertion. Swimming is hard work. It is three to five times more work to swim than it is to walk, and it is significantly more work for a poor swimmer to swim a given distance than it is for a good swimmer to swim the same distance. If you are not a good swimmer or if you have been mainly sedentary, you should not choose swimming as your initial exercise activity. It will be too difficult for you to control your level of exertion so that your pulse rate stays within the desired range.

Competitive sports activities such as tennis, basketball, racquetball, and handball are all excellent dynamic exercise activities. However, until you have reached a fairly high level of physical conditioning, you should not employ a competitive sports activity to improve your level of physical fitness. These are stop and go activities, and unless you are very skilled in a sport it is unlikely that you will be in motion more than about 20 percent of the time. As you will learn later, in order to improve your level of physical fitness, you must sustain your target pulse rate for about 10 to 20 minutes. It is unlikely that you can accomplish this unless you and your partner are both fairly skilled players. Also, *the competitive nature of the activity may present a problem.* If you are not physically fit, it may be hazardous to allow your pulse rate to rise too high. You should remember that blood pressure goes up as pulse rate goes up. If you become too competitive, you may exceed the safe level of pulse rate. Until you have achieved your desired level of physical fitness, you should participate in competitive sports only for relaxed recreational activity.

A program of calisthenics is desirable as *one* part of an exercise program, but it is unrealistic to assume that you will regularly exercise for a sufficient length of time to improve your cardiovascular fitness *unless* you join a supervised program. It may be boring to exercise alone. It may be even more boring to perform calisthenics alone. You have to exercise continually to improve endurance, and it's too easy to stop and rest when you perform calisthenics on your own.

2. The Recommended Method of Performing Dynamic Exercise
You will best protect your blood pressure by keeping your muscles

as relaxed as possible. Tense muscles raise blood pressure. Whatever you do, do it smoothly and naturally. Stay relaxed. It is very important that you *do not get overheated.* Heat is the real enemy of those who exercise. Don't exercise if it is very hot, and do not take a very hot shower, sauna, or steam bath immediately after you exercise. If the weather is very hot, exercise only in the early morning or in the late afternoon or early evening, when the sun is not directly overhead. Wear loose comfortable clothing which allows the air to circulate and the sweat to evaporate.

You already know that when you exercise, your working muscles demand a large amount of blood and your heart must beat more rapidly in order to recirculate the blood and keep the muscles supplied with food and oxygen. In addition, these working muscles create heat, and it is also work for your heart to get rid of this heat. Your body rids itself of heat by circulating the blood close to the surface of the skin so that the heat can be lost to the air. Sweating speeds up this cooling process because the evaporation of sweat cools down the surface of the skin. If the air is warm or humid, sweat evaporates more slowly, and it becomes more difficult for your body to get rid of its excess heat. In order to speed up the heat loss process, the arteries near the surface of the skin will dilate so that a larger amount of blood comes into contact with the skin surface.

Do you see the problem? What happens when arteries dilate? The resistance to the flow of blood goes down, and blood flows more easily through these dilated arteries. Now the heart has another problem. Not only are the arteries to the working muscles dilated and demanding a larger amount of blood, but also the arteries near the surface of the skin are now dilated, and they too are demanding a larger amount of blood. The only way that the heart can cope with this situation is to beat even faster. Eventually, the heart will be unable to supply the muscles with enough food and oxygen while still meeting the body's need to cool off. As the muscles' fuel supply drops off, they will begin to fatigue. They may even develop painful cramps, but this is not the worst of the situation. Remember that during dynamic exercise your blood pressure goes up in order to circulate sufficient blood to the muscles and still make sure that the brain gets all the oxygen it needs. If your body gets too hot, the combination of the dilated arteries to the working muscles and the dilated arteries at the surface of the skin may reduce the resistance to the flow of blood to such a low level that your blood pressure starts to fall. This is *not* a good thing. This fall in the blood pressure endangers the brain. In order to protect the brain, the heart tries to beat even faster to keep the flow of blood going to all the places it has to go. If not corrected, this process can lead to the collapse of the cardiovascular system.

If arteriosclerosis of the coronary arteries is present, the heart may beat so fast that it outruns its own supply of blood, and this can cause a heart attack. (This cannot happen to a heart that has normal coronary arteries). If the fall in blood pressure is severe enough, it may be impossible for sufficient blood to get to the brain, and this may cause you to faint.

No matter which type of dynamic exercise activity you choose, it is extremely important that you not get overheated. Saunas and steam baths make no sense at all. They do no good, and they are potentially dangerous. Physical fitness improves because the muscles which regularly participate in dynamic exercise learn to use food and oxygen more efficiently and consequently the heart does not have to work as hard to supply them as it would unfit muscles. Sitting in a hot room causes the heart to speed up because the arteries near the surface of the skin dilate so that the body can lose heat more rapidly. Your muscles are not working when you sit in a sauna or steam bath. This isolated rapid heart beat in the absence of the rhythmic muscular activity of either the arms or the legs does not lead to an improved level of physical fitness, but it can lead to cardiovascular collapse or a heart attack.

Whatever type of dynamic exercise you choose, you should warm up before you begin the activity and you should cool down after you complete the activity unless you are beginning your program at a low level of physical exercise. For example, if you are beginning with a walking–slow jogging program (and it is strongly recommended that you do), there is no need to warm up or cool down. When you begin to exercise more vigorously, you should spend about 5 to 15 or so minutes getting your body going. There is nothing complicated about this. To warm up you simply engage first in a low level of physical activity before you engage in more vigorous activity. (In the next section you will learn that "vigorous" means the level of physical activity which is required to raise your pulse rate to the target level and hold it there for 10 to 20 minutes.) Obviously, it would be unwise to suddenly jump out of the chair that you are now sitting in and begin immediately to exercise at a rate that will bring your pulse up from its resting level of perhaps 70 beats per minute to say, 160 beats per minute. Your muscles, heart, and lungs need a few minutes to adjust before you undertake this level of activity. All you need to do is walk fast enough to bring your pulse up to perhaps 100 beats per minute for about 5 minutes. It is also of benefit to give your muscles a little warming up by stretching them. Unless you intend to be a runner, there is no need to engage in an elaborate set of stretching exercises; all you need to do is move them about a little. Swing and stretch your arms, tilt your trunk from side to side, bend forward, and stretch your legs. Perform some simple calisthenics, but do not do anything that puts a large curve in your back. For example, don't try to touch your toes with great dedication. All this will accomplish is a sore back, and, if your back is at all unstable, it may aggravate or even precipitate a disc condition. When you get to the point where you wish to be a serious runner or engage in competitive sports at a high level, then you may wish to buy a book that will more specifically instruct you in preliminary stretching exercises.

Cooling down is like warming up. Just as you should not suddenly begin exercising vigorously if you have been not moving at all, neither should you suddenly become immobile when you have been moving vigorously. Remember that the arteries to the working muscles are widely dilated, and there is a lot of blood in these muscles. If you suddenly stop moving them, the blood will tend to stay there and not return to the heart. The heart would like that blood back, because even if your muscles are through with it, your brain still wants its share. If you suddenly stop and either stand in one place or sit down, there may be suddenly too little blood for the brain. Although it is unlikely that you will actually faint, you may feel lightheaded. Remember, too, that the reason the arteries to the working muscles dilate in the first place is because the working muscles release chemicals that force the arteries to do this. To reverse this process, your body has to get rid of these chemicals. The rhythmic contraction and relaxation of muscles pump the blood in the muscles back to the heart. Consequently, once you are through jogging or running vigorously, you should continue walking at a relaxed pace for about 5 minutes so that the blood in the muscles is pumped back up to the heart. If you feel that you absolutely must rest immediately after exercising, then lie down. If you have been swimming vigorously, you should either continue to swim slowly or get out of the water and walk for 5 minutes or so. The same is true if you have been vigorously bicycling or playing a competitive sport.

3. Your Target Heart Rate

Improved physical fitness is achieved by participating in an endurance exercise (dynamic exercise) with sufficient vigor, duration, and regularity that muscles adapt and learn to more efficiently use their food and oxygen. The vigor of the exercise is determined by the speed of the heartbeat. Most experts believe that the speed at which the heart must beat to allow the exercising muscles to adapt to the exercise activity is about 85 percent of the "maximum" pulse rate. This 85 percent is called the *target heart rate*, and it is determined by your age. Earlier it was mentioned that the maximum heart rate that can be achieved naturally goes down as one grows older. Consequently, the older you are, the lower your target pulse rate will be. The older individual makes relatively the same effort as the younger individual: *both will be exercising at about 85 percent of their maximum capability.* A younger individual is simply able to do more physical work at 85 percent of the maximum work capacity than an older person can achieve. Just because the target heart rate is higher for a younger person than for an older person does not mean that the overall benefit of the exercise program is greater for the younger person. Both will achieve the same health benefit. You will *not* gain more by attempting to go beyond your target heart rate. Furthermore, it is potentially dangerous. You will achieve all the benefits of improved cardiovascular fitness by behaving sensibly.

Your maximum heart rate is easy to determine. It is calculated by the following formula:

Your Maximum Heart Rate Is 220 Minus Your Age in Years

For example, if you are 30 years of age, your maximum heart rate is $220 - 30 = 190$. If you are 50, your maximum heart rate is $220 - 50 = 170$.

Your Target Heart Rate Is Also Easy to Determine: It Is Simply 85 Percent of the Maximum Heart Rate

For example, if you are 30 years of age, your maximum heart rate is 190, and your target heart rate is $190 \times 0.85 = 161.5$, or about 162. If you are 50 years of age, your maximum heart rate is 170 and your target heart rate is $170 \times 0.85 = 144.5$ or about 145. The target heart rate is *not* a precise number, and you only have to approximate it.

To save you the bother of performing any calculations, you can determine your target heart rate from this table. You should choose the age closest to your own age. For example, if you are 42, choose 40 in the table. If your age is 43, choose 45 in the table.

TABLE OF TARGET HEART RATES

Age in Years	Maximum Heart Rate	Target Heart Rate
25	195	166
30	190	162
35	185	157
40	180	153
45	175	149
50	170	145
55	165	140
60	160	136
65	155	132
70	150	128
75	145	123
80	140	119

All individuals of the same age have the same target heart rate as long as they do not have any underlying heart disease. (If heart disease is present, the target heart rate should initially be about 40 percent of the maximum heart rate.) Even though two individuals are the same age, it is unlikely that they will require the same degree of physical exertion to reach their target rate. Let's look at age 40. The target heart rate is about 153 beats per minute. A 40-year-old individual who has been exercising regularly may have to jog a mile in, say, nine minutes to get the pulse rate up to this level, but another 40-year-old whose major athletic activity has been eating may achieve this same pulse rate simply by puffing down the street for a block or two. Obviously, one 40-year-old is more physically fit than the other. The more physical effort that you must make before you reach your target pulse rate, the more physically fit you are.

As you become physically fit, you will have to gradually increase the level of your exertion to continue to improve your level of fitness. Your target heart rate stays the same, but as you become more physically fit, it will require a greater absolute effort to get your pulse rate up to the desired level and to keep it there. Perhaps when you begin your fitness program you will choose a walking–jogging–running program. Let's assume your target heart rate is 150 beats per minute. When you first start your program, you may achieve this by brisk walking. If you are faithful to your program, it will not be long before you will have to jog at a moderate speed to get your pulse rate to 150 per minute. Perhaps within a few months you will have actually run to get your pulse rate to this level.

The target heart rate is not a precise number. Most exercise specialists feel that the best results are obtained when you exercise at close to 85 percent of your maximum heart rate, but there are some experts who argue that exercising at as low as 60 percent of your maximum heart rate will still allow you to achieve a high level of physical fitness. Until more data is obtained, it seems best to advise you to use the 85 percent figure. If future studies reveal that a lower figure will do the job, no harm will have resulted because you expended some extra energy. If future studies do prove the 85 percent figure to be correct, you will have been spared the possibility of not achieving your best state of physical fitness.

4. The Duration of Exercise at the Target Heart Rate

You will need to sustain your heartbeat at the target heart rate for about 10 to 20 minutes to improve your level of cardiovascular fitness. For example, if your target heart rate is 150 beats per minutes and you can reach this heart rate by walking briskly, you must continue to walk briskly for 10 to 20 minutes. As your level of fitness improves and you find it necessary to jog or to run to achieve this pulse rate, you will then have to jog or run for 10 or 20 minutes. It is as simple as that. The only problem is trying to measure your pulse rate while you are exercising. This is not easy to do. The best thing to do is to slow down or stop your activity for six seconds so that you can count your pulse, multiply this by ten, and then immediately resume your activity. For example, if you are jogging, stop or slow down to a walk and count your pulse for six seconds. If your target heart rate is 150 beats per minute, then you want to aim for a level of exertion that gives you a count of 15 in six seconds. Absolute precision is not possible and not necessary. Unless you have underlying heart disease or a very serious elevation of your blood pressure, exceeding your target heart rate by a small amount will be of no consequence. Just try to keep within the desired range for the required period of time.

When you first start your program, you may find it necessary to slow down every three minutes or so to check your pulse rate. As your level of physical fitness improves, you will be surprised to see how steadily your pulse rate will hold at a particular level of exertion. Once you are familiar with the degree of effort that it requires to get your pulse rate to the desired level, you will be able to exercise safely without counting your pulse rate at all.

5. The Frequency of the Exercise Program

Three or four exercise periods a week are recommended. There is nothing wrong with exercising more frequently than this, but studies suggest that you will not improve cardiovascular fitness if you exercise less frequently.

6. Making Progress

You now know that the more of an effort that you must make to reach your target pulse rate, the more fit is your cardiovascular system. You will have no difficulty recognizing that you have made progress, because improved cardiovascular fitness means improved endurance. You will know that your endurance has improved because activities that once caused fatigue and breathlessness you will now be able to perform with relative ease. However, you should understand that at every stage of your exercise program, you will be working hard. To exercise at 85 percent of your maximum capacity is *always* hard work. When you first start your program, you may find that 10 to 20 minutes of brisk walking is hard work. If it is not hard work, it will not lead to improved cardiovascular fitness! Later in your program, you may have to jog at a moderately rapid pace to experience the same feeling of hard work. Progress is made by gradually increasing the intensity of your effort as your ability to exercise improves.

You should not rush your program. If you have been very sedentary, you may find it just too difficult to maintain a level of physical activity which keeps your pulse rate at 85 percent of maximum even for 10 minutes. You may need to start at 60 percent of maximum and slowly build up to 85 percent. You should plan to devote about *six months* to becoming physically fit. Remember that your goal is to engage in some form of dynamic exercise activity that allows you to sustain your target pulse rate for 10 to 20 minutes and that you will do this three or four times per week. You should not try to increase your level of exertion more often than about every two to three weeks. You should get used to one level of exertion and feel comfortable with it before you try to do more.

How much progress should you make? There is no real answer to this question but it seems most sensible to work diligently on your program for about six months and then maintain the progress you have made by choosing a level of effort and types of activity that you find enjoyable. If your daily activities usually keep your pulse rate in the range of 70 to 90 beats per minute and you improve your cardiovascular fitness so that you can sustain your target heart rate for 10 to 20 minutes without undue fatigue, you have probably achieved all that you need to achieve.

7. Maintaining Your State of Improved Cardiovascular Fitness

If you have been fairly sedentary, it is suggested that you begin with a walking–jogging–running program. This is the easiest program to follow, for the reasons mentioned earlier, and it is easier for you to measure your progress with this than with any other form of dynamic exercise. Once you have improved your fitness level, that is, after you have devoted about six months to your program, you can then engage in other activities in order to *maintain* the level of fitness that you have achieved. You can now begin to consider other kinds of dynamic activities that will allow you to sustain your target pulse rate for the required 10 to 20 minutes. Swimming, bicycling, hiking, cross-country skiing, tennis, racquetball, and other competitive sports activities are now appropriate for you. The only requirement is that you acquire the skill to participate in such an activity with sufficient intensity to achieve and sustain your target pulse rate. You cannot maintain any improved level of physical fitness unless you continue to exercise regularly, so it is very important for you to choose activities which you enjoy and which you look forward to performing.

8. Changing From One Type of Physical Activity to Another

If you have employed one type of physical activity to improve your level of physical fitness, it is safe for you to use another type of physical activity for exercise as long as *both types of exercise use the same muscles*. For example, if you have been walking–jogging–running, you can safely assume that you can bicycle with the same intensity and not dangerously elevate your blood pressure.

Endurance training is best achieved by regularly exercising the leg muscles, and this is what has been recommended to you. You should remember that one of the major reasons that regular exercise improves cardiovascular fitness is that the muscles which are regularly exercised adapt. They learn how to use their supply of food and oxygen more efficiently, so your heart has to perform less work to supply them with blood. However, you *cannot* suddenly decide to perform an activity that requires the vigorous use of your arm muscles if you have been regularly using your leg muscles to improve your state of cardiovascular fitness. For example, vigorous swimming or rowing should not be performed. The muscles of your arms will not have achieved the same level of improved food and oxygen utilization as your leg muscles, and your heart will suddenly be challenged with an unusually high work load. Under this circumstance, your blood pressure and your heart may not be protected.

Even when you are in good physical condition, you should still avoid strenuous isometric activities, for these activities will still result in a substantial rise in blood pressure during the time that the muscles are held in fixed contraction.

9. Blood Pressure Medications and Exercise
Blood pressure medicines do not protect you and can be dangerous if they prevent the normal rise in blood pressure which MUST occur when you exercise vigorously. You know that your blood pressure must go up when you engage in a vigorous dynamic physical activity. When you are briskly walking, for example, there is a large increase in the flow of blood to the working muscles of the legs. To compensate for this, the nervous system delivers the message, "Raise the blood pressure," to the arteries in the arms and the abdomen; these arteries constrict, the heart rate goes up, and blood pressure goes up. Since many medicines that are used to treat high blood pressure work by interfering with the message, "Raise the blood pressure," you can see the problem. If a blood pressure medicine is so powerful that the arteries to the arms and the abdomen are unable to respond to the message and do not constrict, the sudden diversion of blood to the working muscles of the legs will result in a sudden serious drop in blood pressure, which will deprive the brain of its oxygen supply. The result is anything from a feeling of lightheadedness to loss of consciousness (fainting), depending upon the degree of the drop in blood pressure.

Fortunately, most blood pressure medicines are not sufficiently powerful to prevent the diversion of blood away from your arms and abdomen when you engage in vigorous dynamic exercise with your legs. The signal from the nervous system is so strong that it gets out of the nervous system and to the receptors in the arteries despite the presence of blood pressure medication. However, many doctors agree that one medication, guanethidine and related compounds, is so strong that it is definitely hazardous if you are exercising vigorously. A few others are strong enough to be potentially hazardous. Some medications, although not necessarily dangerous to you when you are exercising, will impair your ability to exercise because they will cause you to fatigue more easily. Little is known about the potential hazards of combinations of medications during vigorous dynamic exercise, and in certain circumstances the only way that you will be able to determine whether or not your own treatment program can result in a dangerous drop in your blood pressure when you exercise will be to undergo an exercise stress test while you are taking your medications.

The medicines will be discussed in the same order that they were discussed in Chapter 7.

Medicines That Interrupt the Message in the Nervous System

clonidine Of all the drugs which work by interrupting the message in the nervous system, clonidine is one of the safest to use if you wish to engage in vigorous physical activity. Although the studies are not extensive, those that have been performed indicate that blood pressure does rise during dynamic exercise and that dynamic exercise is safely performed in the presence of clonidine.

guanethidine and related compounds It may be very dangerous to engage in vigorous or dynamic activity if you are taking guanethidine or related compounds. Even brisk walking can cause a serious drop in blood pressure. Unless you take an exercise stress test and prove that your blood pressure responds appropriately to exercise, *do not* exercise vigorously when you take any of these medicines.

methyldopa Methyldopa is almost, but probably not quite as safe as clonidine. An occasional individual who takes this medication will experience a drop in blood pressure while exercising. Usually the fall in blood pressure is small, and there seems to be little danger that your blood pressure will significantly fall during dynamic exercise while you are taking this medication.

prazosin Vigorous dynamic exercise may cause your blood pressure to fall too low if you are taking prazosin. Unless you undergo an exercise stress test and prove that you can exercise vigorously while taking this medication, you should assume that vigorous exercise is potentially hazardous.

Rauwolfia compounds such as reserpine It is safe to exercise vigorously while you are taking reserpine and other Rauwolfia compounds.

Medicines That Prevent a Blood Pressure Machine From Receiving a Signal

propranolol and other beta-blockers Propranolol and the other beta-blockers are safe to use during dynamic exercise. They seldom cause a serious drop in blood pressure during exercise. However, these medications have the property of preventing the heart from beating as rapidly as it would beat if you were not taking the medication. Since vigorous exercise requires a rapid heartbeat, you may not be able to exercise either as vigorously or as long when you take a beta-blocker. There is no danger in this, but you should know that these medicines may limit your exercise capacity. You should also remember that they have the property of bringing out underlying lung disease. Since lung diseases such as asthma, emphysema, and chronic bronchitis limit exercise ability, you may find your ability to exercise reduced even further if you have lung disease and take one of these medicines. In this regard, many of the newer beta-blockers are safer than propranolol, but it is best to avoid these medicines altogether if you have lung problems now or once suffered from asthma. Some of the beta-blockers have more of a tendency to produce muscle fatigue than others. If you are taking a beta-blocker and find that your ability to exercise seems impaired because of leg fatigue, ask your doctor either to substitute another beta-blocker or to switch you to a different class of medication.

Medicines That Take Over the Control of a Blood Pressure Machine

Diuretics As long as you do not become dehydrated, it should be safe for you to participate in vigorous dynamic exercise while you are taking any of the diuretics. It will be important for you to be sure that your potassium level is within the range of normal. During normal everyday activities, a moderate lowering of potassium is usually considered safe. However, any vigorous exercise activity can cause irregularities of the heartbeat, and a low potassium level potentiates the development of heartbeat irregularities. Thus, the combination of a low potassium and vigorous dynamic exercise may be hazardous. This is a time when the use of either a potassium supplement or a potassium-sparing agent may prove beneficial.

As long as you do not exercise when it is very hot, you should be able to avoid dehydration. On a hot day you can lose a great deal of water even though you do not sweat. It is especially important to avoid exercising in the direct sun or in extreme heat. You should, of course, maintain an adequate fluid intake. Unless you feel weak or lightheaded, you should not take extra salt. Water or other unsalted liquids should adequately replace the liquid you lose from perspiring.

hydralazine and dihydrallazine Even though hydralazine and dihydrallazine are medicines that work to directly dilate arteries, it is generally safe to participate in dynamic exercise while you are taking either medication. No special precautions seem necessary.

minoxidil There is little information about this potent new medicine. Because it is so potent, you should consider it unsafe to exercise vigorously while you are taking it unless you undergo an exercise stress test.

calcium antagonists There is too little information to make a recommendation about this new group of medicines.

Combinations of Medicines
Medical scientists have not extensively studied the effect that high blood pressure medications have on individuals who engage in vigorous exercise. Most of the studies have involved only a few subjects taking only a single medicine. The information regarding the effect of single medicines is scant, and the information regarding combinations of medicine is practically nonexistent. With the renewed interest in exercise and the increasing awareness that participation in a regular exercise program is beneficial not only to those with normal blood pressure but also to those who have high blood pressure, perhaps more work will be done in the future. The safety of exercise for those who take high blood pressure medications is a neglected area of medical investigation, and more studies are urgently needed. The following information should be considered as a generally accurate guideline for you to follow, but you should be aware that the available data are not extensive.

The Combination of a Diuretic and One Other Medicine
Clonidine, probably as safe as clonidine alone.

Guanethidine and related compounds, probably even more

dangerous than guanethidine alone. Be very careful.

Methyldopa, probably as safe as methyldopa alone. If you are taking large doses of methyldopa (two grams a day or more), it may be best to take a stress test.

Prazosin, probably even more dangerous than prazosin alone. Be very careful.

Reserpine, probably as safe as reserpine alone.

Propranolol and other beta-blockers, probably as safe as either medicine alone.

Hydralazine, probably as safe as hydralazine alone.

Minoxidil, in the face of too little information, wisest to forego vigorous dynamic activity while taking this unless you have had a stress test.

The Combination of a Diuretic and Two Other Medicines There is not enough information to give you safe advice. The following combinations are probably safe:

Diuretic plus beta-blocker plus hydralazine
Diuretic plus reserpine plus hydralazine

Other Combinations of Medicines The combination of beta-blocker plus hydralazine is probably safe.

SUMMARY

A regular program of dynamic exercise at some level is safe if you have high blood pressure, and there are many benefits to such a program. If you have mild high blood pressure, regular exercise may produce a permanent lowering of your blood pressure. (Scientists are still unsure how this good result is accomplished. It may be that the vascular resistance in the arteries of the legs is permanently lowered.) If you improve your level of cardiovascular fitness you will be able to perform more physical activity with less strain on your heart; this may lessen the likelihood of your developing future heart disease and it may improve the function of your heart if you already have heart disease. Regular dynamic exercise usually causes a loss of weight, and this is another way in which it may lead to a lowering of your blood pressure. If you begin your exercise program slowly and use your pulse rate as a guide, there is little danger to you.

Perhaps the major hazard comes from the blood pressure medicines themselves. It is important that your blood pressure be allowed to go up when you engage in vigorous dynamic exercise. If you are taking a very potent medication (such as guanethidine) or a combination of medications, vigorous exercise may cause your blood pressure to fall during the time that you are exercising. You can determine whether your medicines allow you to exercise safely by taking an exercise stress test.

Isometric exercise should generally be avoided. This form of exercise requires muscles to be held in fixed contraction, and this may cause a large rise in blood pressure during the exercise activity. You should exercise with a natural rhythm and keep your muscles as relaxed as possible. You should not exercise if it is excessively hot, and you should not take a very hot shower, a steam bath, or a sauna immediately after you exercise.

15

HOW TO CHOOSE AND USE YOUR OWN BLOOD PRESSURE MEASUREMENT KIT

Before reading these instructions, it is suggested that you reread the material presented in Chapters 1 through 3. These chapters fully explained the general principles of blood pressure measurement. A review of this information should make it easier for you to learn to measure your own blood pressure.

This section is divided into three parts. First, the general principles of blood pressure measurement are briefly summarized. Then information is presented to help you purchase your own blood pressure kit. Finally, step-by-step instructions are given to help you use your equipment so that you can easily and accurately measure your own blood pressure.

A BRIEF REVIEW

A blood pressure measurement consists of two numbers. The top number, the systolic blood pressure, is the pressure during the systolic phase of heart contraction. This is the pressure in the arteries when the full force of the contracting heart is pushing upon the bloodstream. The bottom number, the diastolic pressure, is the pressure during the diastolic phase of heart contraction. This is the pressure in the arteries between heartbeats while the heart is filling up with blood.

The systolic blood pressure reflects the maximum force which is required for the heart to circulate blood to all parts of the body in order to deliver food and oxygen and to remove the waste products of tissue metabolism. The diastolic pressure reflects the elastic tension in the arterial walls. It is the force with which the elastic walls of the arteries press upon the blood to keep all parts of the body in contact with blood between heartbeats. This contact ensures that blood does not leave your feet when you stand on your head or leave your head when you stand on your feet.

If you stand by the side of a stream, how can you tell if the water is flowing if you are unable to either see or touch the water in the stream? You can *hear* the flow of the water. As long as there is a rock or a branch in the stream to create a source of turbulence, the movement of the flowing water will create rippling sounds. By listening for these sounds, you can decide whether or not the water is flowing. If the flow of water is very slow or if the rock or branch is very small, the sounds may be very soft. In this case, you may have to use some sort of listening device to amplify the sounds so that your ears can detect them. This is how blood pressure is measured.

Blood pressure is measured by standing by the side of the blood stream and listening to the flow of blood while at the same time watching a pressure gauge. Both your eyes and your ears are necessary. In order to hear the flow of the blood stream, you must place a rock into the stream to create a source of turbulence. You create a "rock" by wrapping a blood pressure cuff around your arm and raising the pressure so that the cuff squeezes on the artery and indents its wall. The indentation of the wall becomes a source of turbulence, and tapping sounds are heard as the blood streams by. The tapping sounds are very soft, and to hear these "blood pressure" sounds some sort of listening device is required: therefore, a stethoscope or a microphone is placed over the artery. The stethoscope amplifies the sounds and delivers them directly to your ears. The microphone converts the sounds into electronic signals which can then be fed either into an amplifier and speaker so that you can hear the tapping sounds without a stethoscope (as a series of beeps) or into a light source so that you can "see" the tapping sounds (as series of flashing lights).

The top or systolic blood pressure number is measured by raising the pressure in the blood pressure cuff high enough to completely squeeze the artery shut. Now blood cannot flow, and no sounds can be heard. The pressure in the cuff is now slowly reduced while carefully watching the pressure gauge. When the very first tapping blood pressure sound appears, the number which registers on the pressure gauge is noted. This is the systolic blood pressure. The systolic blood pressure is the maximum pressure with which the heart must push on the blood stream to force blood through the tiny opening that you have created. At first the tapping sounds are relatively loud, because the "rock" in the flowing stream is relatively large. As the pressure in the cuff is gradually lowered, the indentation of the arterial wall lessens, and the sounds become softer. Eventually, the wall of the artery is no longer indented at all, and the blood pressure sounds disappear. The number which is noted on the pressure gauge just when the last sound is heard is the diastolic blood pressure. This is the elastic tension of the arterial wall, and it is the pressure with which the artery pushes on the blood between heart beats.

It is relatively easy to measure systolic blood pressure, and it is also relatively easy to understand the principle of its measurement. Not so with diastolic pressure. It is more difficult to measure diastolic pressure, because the technique makes it necessary to note the reading on the pressure gauge just when the sound disappears. It is necessary to listen for the *absence* of a sound, and this requires more practice than listening for the appearance of a sound. It is also more difficult to understand how the disappearance of the blood pressure sound can represent the diastolic blood pressure. The following experiment will help to make this clear: Stretch a rubber band between the fingers of one hand. Now take a pencil in your other hand and press in upon a section of the rubber band so that you deform its wall. You know when you have applied enough pressure to indent the wall of the rubber band because you can see the deformity. If you close your eyes, you can still detect the deformity by rubbing your finger along the inside of the rubber band. But how can you detect the indentation if you are unable to either see it or feel it? One way to accomplish this is to use the same technique that is used to measure blood pressure. Pretend that water flows along the inside of the rubber band. When you push on the rubber band with your pencil and indent its wall, you can imagine that you hear the turbulence as the imaginary water flows past the deformity. You are now ready to measure the "diastolic" pressure of your rubber band system.

Connect your pencil to an imaginary "pencil pressure" gauge and push in on the rubber band with your pencil until you imagine that you hear the "pencil pressure" sounds produced as the imaginary water flows by the indentation. Now slowly reduce the pressure with which your pencil pushes in on the rubber band while you watch your imaginary gauge. Note the number which registers on the pressure gauge just when the last imaginary sound is heard. This is the elastic tension of the wall of the rubber band. It is the "diastolic pressure" of your rubber band system.

To measure blood pressure accurately, you should use the arm which gives the highest reading. Except under unusual circumstances, the blood pressure cuff goes on the upper right arm, because blood pressure is almost always higher in the right arm. The cuff is made of a nonstretchable cloth which covers a rubber bladder similar to a balloon. Two tubes are connected to the bladder. One tube brings air from a rubber squeeze bulb into the bladder to pump it up and create pressure. The other tube con-

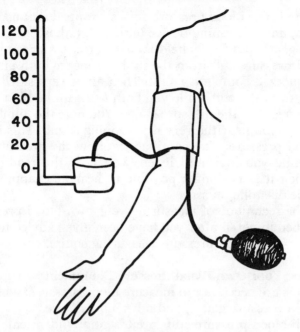

Mercury pressure gauge (Mercury manometer)

nects the bladder to a pressure gauge, and this allows you to know the pressure inside the blood pressure cuff at all times.

The *standard* blood pressure gauge is the mercury manometer. This is simply a vertical glass tube immersed within a small glass reservoir of liquid mercury. A tube connects the rubber bladder of the blood pressure cuff to the glass reservoir. When air is pumped into the bladder from the rubber squeeze bulb, it simultaneously goes to the pressure gauge. As the air which is pumped into the blood pressure cuff pushes on the tissues to squeeze the artery, it also pushes on the liquid mercury and forces it to rise in the vertical glass tube. The height to which the liquid column of mercury rises in the tube is the blood pressure.

The units of blood pressure are millimeters of mercury. The glass tube of the pressure gauge has a series of lines etched upon it, and each line represents 1 millimeter. If the blood pressure is recorded as "140 over 80," this means that the first sound was heard when the mercury was at the 140 millimeter mark and that the last sound was heard when the mercury was at the 80 millimeter mark. Millimeter is abbreviated mm, and mercury is abbreviated Hg, which is the chemical symbol for mercury. "140 over 80" means that the systolic blood pressure is 140 mm Hg and that the diastolic blood pressure is 80 mm Hg. Rather than write "over," a slash is used: "140/80" means "140 over 80."

The technique of blood pressure measurement is quite uncomplicated. The blood pressure cuff is wrapped around the upper right arm, and a listening device (either a stethoscope or a microphone) is gently but firmly held over the artery. Air is pumped into the blood pressure cuff from the rubber squeeze bulb until the artery is squeezed completely shut. Then air is very slowly allowed to escape from the cuff while you both *listen* to the blood pressure sounds and *look* at the pressure gauge. You note the number on the gauge when you hear the very first tapping sound. This is the systolic blood pressure. You continue to allow the pressure to drop slowly while you look and listen. You note the reading on the gauge when it is no longer possible to hear any tapping sounds. This is the diastolic pressure.

The technique of measuring your own blood pressure will be described in detail after you have been given advice to help you select your own blood pressure measuring equipment.

Purchasing Your Own Blood Pressure Equipment
Three items are necessary to measure blood pressure: a blood pressure cuff, a pressure gauge, and a listening device.

All blood pressure cuffs are essentially identical. There are two features, however, which are very desirable, a D-ring and a Velcro lock, and if possible you should select a cuff that has these additions. More about the importance of these special features later in the chapter.

There are three types of pressure gauges: the mercury manometer, the mechanical aneroid manometer, and the electronic aneroid manometer. The *mercury manometer* is the standard of accuracy. It is not only the most accurate and the most reliable gauge, but it is also usually the least expensive. This type of gauge is highly recommended. It should cost between $15 and $40. The *mechanical aneroid gauge* is usually slightly more expensive than the mercury gauge, and it is less reliable. The aneroid manometer replaces the liquid mercury with springs; it looks like a clock that has only one hand. If you purchase a mechanical aneroid gauge, you will have to have it checked initially against a mercury gauge and should continue checking it at regular intervals. If it is dropped or bounced around a great deal, it may either break altogether or become inaccurate. A mechanical aneroid gauge should cost between $18 and $40. The *electronic aneroid gauges* are the most expensive. They always come with an electronic microphone. The reason to purchase an electronic gauge is *not* for the gauge. The gauge is not as reliable as the mercury gauge, must be checked against the mercury gauge at regular intervals, and is rather fragile. It probably will break if it is dropped. The electronic gauge is purchased because of the *microphone*. The microphone detects the sound and either sends it to a speaker so that you can hear it, or to

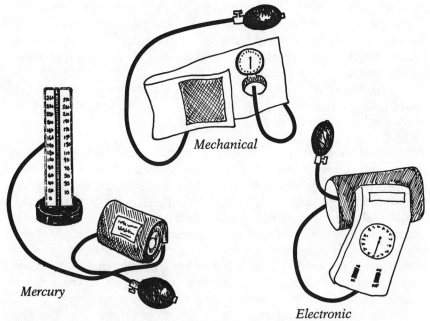

Mechanical

Mercury

Electronic

The three types of pressure gauges

a light so that you can see it, or both. The electronic gauge is purchased for convenience of operation, and not because it is more reliable or more accurate than the other two types of pressure gauges. Do not allow the flashing lights and/or musical beeps of the electronic instruments to influence you. The very best blood pressure measuring device is the simple inexpensive mercury manometer. *Only* if you have trouble learning to hear with the stethoscope should you consider going to the added expense of buying an electronic device. They run from $70 to as much as $200.

Unless you purchase an electronic device, you will need a stethoscope. Stethoscopes are not expensive. If purchased separately, it should not cost more than $2 to $3. The desirable features of a stethoscope will be discussed later.

Usually home blood pressure measuring instruments are sold as kits. They can be obtained at medical supply houses, pharmacies, and department stores. A typical kit will include either a mercury manometer plus a blood pressure cuff plus a stethoscope, or it will include a mechanical aneroid manometer plus a blood pressure cuff plus a stethoscope. It is *not* necessary to buy all three as a single purchase. In fact it usually is more desirable not to do so. Blood pressure cuffs and pressure gauges are interchangeable. You can use *any* blood pressure cuff with *any* mercury or mechanical aneroid gauge. Few of the existing kits are entirely satisfactory; you will get the best equipment by selecting the cuff and the manometer *separately*. This way you can be assured that each has the features which are most desirable for self-determination of blood pressure. As you will soon learn, many of the stethoscopes included with the kits are undesirable, and this is another item which may be best purchased separately.

If you decide to buy an electronic device, you will not have the option of interchanging parts. Electronic instruments must be purchased as a complete package.

The Blood Pressure Cuff All blood pressure cuffs have approximately the same construction. A rubber bladder is encased within a nonstretchable cloth cover. The rubber bladder occupies the entire width of the cuff ("width" means the distance between your elbow and your shoulder) but only about one-fourth of the length of the cuff ("length" means the distance around your arm). It is extremely important that you choose a cuff that is both the correct length *and* the correct width for your arm. Although the cloth cover must go around the entire arm at least once, the rubber bladder should not be so long that it can be wrapped upon itself. The cuff should be wide enough to cover about two-thirds of the upper arm between the elbow and the shoulder.

If the cuff is too narrow for your arm, you will get a falsely high reading for both numbers. If the cuff is too wide for your arm, you will get a falsely low reading for both numbers. If the rubber bladder in the cuff is so long that it overlaps itself when wrapped around the arm, falsely low readings will be obtained.

Most adults will need the "standard" size cuff. The standard cuff contains a bladder which is 12 to 13 cm wide (about 5 inches). If you have a very large arm, you may need the "thigh" cuff. This cuff contains a bladder which is 33 to 35 cm wide (about 13 to 14 inches). A "large" adult cuff is also available; this is in between the regular cuff and the thigh cuff in size. If you are purchasing the cuff to take a child's blood pressure or if you have an extremely thin arm, you may need to purchase a cuff that has a 9 cm wide bladder. Most children between the ages of 4 and 8 will need this smaller cuff. Older children usually can use the standard cuff. (It is not recommended that you attempt to measure the blood pressure of a child less than 4 years of age.) If you are in doubt as to which cuff to purchase, ask your physician.

Do not purchase a blood pressure cuff that you cannot return. You will want your doctor to check the cuff to be sure that it is the proper size for your arm or for your child's arm. If it is either too large or too small, you will want to be able to return it.

Measuring your own blood pressure is a *one-handed* operation. Even under the best of circumstances, it requires some dexterity. The arm upon which you place the cuff must be kept relaxed and still. Except in rare circumstances, this will be the *right* arm. Therefore, not only is blood pressure measurement a one-handed operation, it is usually a left-handed operation! Since most individuals are right-handed, this is an added difficulty. The cuff must be placed upon the arm, properly positioned, and made firm all with the left hand. For this reason, it is important not only that you choose a cuff that is the correct size for your arm, but also that you choose one that is properly designed for one-handed operation.

One-handed operation of the blood pressure cuff is greatly facilitated by the presence of both a D-ring and a Velcro lock. Most modern cuffs have the Velcro lock, but many lack the D-ring. The D-ring is also called the *slide-bar*. It is a metal ring which is sewn into the cuff, and it gives you something to pull against when you are trying to firm up the cuff on your arm. If you are not convinced of the importance of a D-ring, try tightening up a blood pressure cuff on your arm without one!

It is important to know that most of the kits on the market include a mercury manometer but do not include a D-ring on the cuff. This is unfortunate, because these are the most accurate and least expensive blood pressure measuring kits. Only the manufacturers who make the more expensive kits seem to have thought to include the D-ring. It is strongly recommended that you ask the

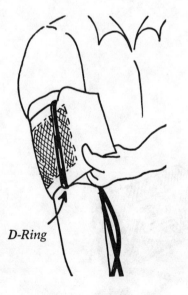

D-Ring

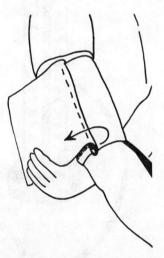

Flip cuff over D-ring and fasten Velcro

company to have a D-ring sewn onto the cuff for you or to substitute a cuff with a D-ring for the one that comes with the kit. Any cuff can be substituted for any other cuff. If you are insistent enough, you should be able to get what you want.

The release valve at the base of the squeeze bulb is a critical element of the blood pressure cuff (see Figure 6). Air both enters and leaves the rubber bladder in the cuff through this valve. When the control knob is closed, air enters the bladder but cannot escape. This allows you to raise the pressure in the cuff by repeatedly squeezing the rubber bulb to pump air into the cuff. A slight turn of the release valve should allow air to *slowly* escape from the cuff. The pressure should drop slowly and evenly. It should not fall more rapidly than 2 to 3 mm Hg per second. *This is slow.* If your blood pressure is 140/80, then the first sound is heard at 140 mm Hg and the last sound is heard at 80 mm Hg. The 60 mm Hg between 140 and 80 is just a little over two inches, and it should take about *30 seconds* for the mercury to fall over this short distance.

Thus when you purchase your cuff, be certain that the squeeze bulb has a good control valve. If you are unable to adjust it easily so that the pressure falls at the desired rate, do not buy it. If you have difficulty adjusting the control knob because of arthri-

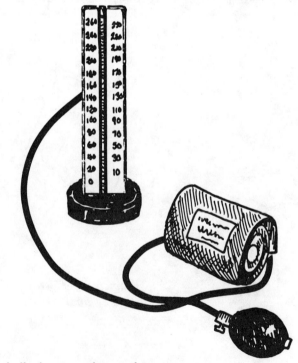

Squeeze bulb showing release valve

tis in your hands, you can purchase a squeeze bulb that has an automatic deflating valve. Unfortunately, few of the existing kits with a mercury pressure gauge possess an automatic deflating valve. This is an oversight on the part of the companies that sell these kits. Many of the kits with mechanical anaeroid manometers offer this convenience, and all of the electronic kits have some sort of an automatic deflating valve. Again, since blood pressure equipment is interchangeable, you should be able to arrange to purchase both a mercury manometer as well as an automatic deflating valve.

The Pressure Gauge The most accurate and reliable pressure gauge is the mercury manometer. Unless you drop it and break its glass tubing, it will always remain accurate. All that is required is that you keep it clean so that the air vents in the glass tubing do not become clogged. If you travel a great deal and wish to carry your blood pressure kit with you, you will have to make sure that your mercury manometer has both a good carrying case and a switch which keeps the mercury from leaking out of the reservoir when the manometer is not in use. There is still the possibility of the glass breaking if your suitcase is bounced around a lot, and this may be one time when a mechanical aneroid gauge should be selected.

An aneroid mechanical pressure gauge is not as reliable as a mercury gauge. It must be checked against a mercury gauge at intervals. If it is inaccurate, you will have to send it back to the company for adjustment. If you drop a mechanical aneroid gauge, it is very likely to become inaccurate, if it continues to work at all. Sometimes, it is very difficult to tell when a gauge has lost its accuracy. If you begin to get blood pressure readings that are very different from your usual ones, have your doctor check your blood pressure with a mercury manometer as well as with your manometer.

Electronic aneroid manometers are not purchased because of the pressure gauge. They are purchased because they contain the microphone which makes using a stethoscope unnecessary. They are purchased for *convenience* rather than accuracy. An electronic gauge should be purchased only if you cannot learn to use a stethoscope. Electronic gauges are sensitive. If bounced around or dropped, they will usually either become inaccurate or break altogether. You should arrange to have an electronic device checked at regular intervals. Your doctor can do this by comparing the reading of your instrument against the reading of a mercury manometer. If your electronic aneroid manometer becomes inaccurate, you will have to send it back to the company for repair.

The Stethoscope A stethoscope is the least expensive item you need to purchase. (Of course, if you purchase an electronic device, you won't need a stethoscope at all.) Usually, a stethoscope comes as part of the blood pressure kit, but often the design of the stethoscopes in these kits is unsatisfactory. The working part of a stethoscope is its *head*. This is the part which is held over the artery to pick up the tapping sounds. The head may be shaped like a bell or funnel or it may be flat and about the size of a half-dollar. The flat type of stethoscope head is called a *diaphragm*. Bell or funnel shaped heads are more difficult to use than the diaphragm type, and they are not recommended even though blood pressure sounds are said to be a little louder with these types.

The earpieces of all stethoscopes are interchangeable. They are simply small round pieces of plastic that screw on to the metal tubing. If the earpieces are too small, they will protrude too far into your ear canals. This situation is both uncomfortable and unnecessary. Try your stethoscope before you buy it. If the earpieces hurt your ears, ask the salesperson to replace them with a larger size. Many of the complete blood pressure kits do not give you a choice of earpieces. If you buy your blood pressure kit through the mail, first ascertain that the stethoscope has not only a flat head but also more than one pair of earpieces. You should have the option of replacing the existing earpieces with larger ones.

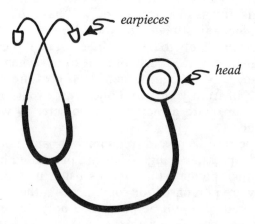

earpieces

head

Electronic Blood Pressure Kits Electronic blood pressure kits are purchased for convenience of operation. These are not as reliable as mercury manometers, and they are fairly delicate. The only reason to purchase one of these expensive instruments is if you have patiently tried to learn to use a stethoscope and have failed.

Not every electronic blood pressure device will work for everyone. These instruments have a built-in microphone. It is essential that the placement of the microphone in the cuff be correct for your arm. An instrument might give perfectly accurate readings on one person's arm and very inaccurate readings on another person's arm. There is no way that you can tell in advance whether the device in which you are interested will work for you. *Do not buy any electronic blood pressure kit that you cannot return.* Take it to your doctor's office and have your pressure checked with this instrument as well as with a mercury manometer. Unles the readings are quite close (within 5 mm Hg), do not buy the instrument.

Summary

1. Buy a cuff that is the correct size for your arm.
2. Buy a cuff that has both a D-ring and a Velcro lock.
3. Make sure that there is a good release valve on the squeeze bulb.
4. Buy a stethoscope with a flat (diaphragm) head and comfortable earpieces.
5. Unless you do a great deal of traveling or cannot learn to use a stethoscope, buy a mercury manometer.
6. If you purchase either a mechanical aneroid manometer or an electronic aneroid manometer, have your doctor check it for accuracy right away.
7. Do not buy any equipment that you cannot return within a given period.

The Technique of Measuring Your Own Blood Pressure

In addition to adequate equipment, measuring your own blood pressure requires three things: patience, a quiet room, and a support for your arm.

Patience Learning to measure your own blood pressure requires practice. It takes time to learn to manipulate the cuff with only one hand. It also takes time to become familiar with the soft tapping blood pressure sounds that you hear through the stethoscope. Keep your blood pressure measuring sessions brief. Practice no more than ten minutes twice a day. Brief practice sessions will keep you from becoming frustrated. Almost everyone can learn to measure blood pressure accurately within about two weeks. Don't try to rush things and don't give up too soon. Do not try too hard at any one session. Relax. Your ears must learn to recognize the tapping blood pressure sounds, and you cannot force them. Brief daily sessions will work best.

A Quiet Room The tapping blood pressure sounds are reasonably soft, and you need a quiet environment which is free of distractions. Since both your eyes and your ears are necessary, the TV set should be switched off. Turning down the volume is not enough.

A Support for Your Arm You can best measure your blood pressure when you are sitting or standing. Your outstretched arm should be supported so that it is about even with the middle of your chest. The ordinary kitchen or dining room table and chair is an ideal support when you are seated. A shelf or counter top will work when you are standing. It is possible to measure your own blood pressure when you are lying down but this is more difficult.

Step-by-Step Instructions 1. Sit or stand quietly for at least five minutes before you measure your blood pressure. Brisk walking, running, step climbing, and carrying bundles can all cause a temporary rise in blood pressure.

2. Place the stethoscope loosely around your neck and let it hang freely. Place the remainder of your equipment on the table or other arm support before you.

3. Sit or stand so that your right forearm and hand can rest comfortably upon a steady support which is about midchest in height.

4. Remove any clothing from the right arm so that both the cuff and the stethoscope can be applied directly to the skin.

5. Slip the blood pressure cuff on your right upper arm and secure it so that it fits fairly snugly. Make sure the control knob of the release valve at the base of the squeeze bulb is open. The bottom edge of the cuff should be an inch or two above the elbow. Most cuffs have a mark near the bottom edge. The cuff should be rotated so that this mark is approximately in line with the brachial artery in the crook of your arm. Proper position of the cuff becomes especially important if the cuff has either a built-in stethoscope or microphone. For instructions on locating the brachial artery, see Step 12 below and also Item 3 of "Problems."

6. Place your outstretched right forearm comfortably on the support in front of you so that all of your arm from the elbow down is supported. Your right hand should be turned so that the palm faces upward.

7. Retighten the cuff so that it does not slip on your arm, and, if necessary, reposition it so that the mark is in the correct place. See Step 12 below and also Item 3 of "Problems."

8. Close the control knob of the release valve.

9. Position the pressure gauge in front of you so that you can easily see the numbers on the gauge.

10. Position the stethoscope earpieces into your ears with your left hand. If you find it difficult to place the earpieces into your ears with one hand, you can place the stethoscope into your ears before you retighten the cuff (Step 7).

There are two methods of proceeding from this point. The object is to be able to pump up the cuff with the squeeze bulb while you simultaneously feel the pulsations of the artery. You want to continue pumping air into the cuff until the pulsations in the artery completely disappear. Method 11a to 14a shows you how to do this using only your left hand. Method 11b to 14b shows you how to do this using both hands. Try both methods, and then choose the one that you find more comfortable.

11a. Place the squeeze bulb in the palm of your left hand and hold it so that you can squeeze it easily by pressing on it with only your thumb and last three fingers. The bulb fits easily into your palm, and it should be easy to repeatedly squeeze it without using your index finger.

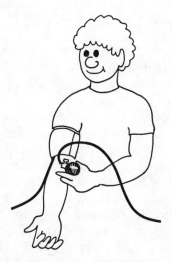

Illustration of method 11a to 14a (left hand only)

11b. Place the squeeze bulb in your right hand and hold it so that you can easily squeeze it and keep the remainder of your right arm reasonably still.

12a. Place the first finger of the left hand on the brachial artery so that you can feel it pulsating. The brachial artery is located just below the junction of the upper arm and the forearm and slightly to the left of center. If you look closely at this part of

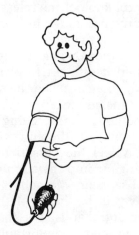

Illustration of method 11b to 14b (both hands)

your arm, often you can see the slight rhythmic lifting up of the skin which lies directly above the artery.

12b. Place the first and second fingers of the right hand on the brachial artery so that you can feel it pulsating. (For instructions on locating the brachial artery, see 12a.)

If you are using electronic equipment, it is still a good idea to follow Steps 12 and 13. They will give you added confidence that your equipment is functioning properly.

13a. Pump up the pressure in the cuff with your left hand and at the same time feel the pulse of the brachial artery with your left index finger until you can no longer feel the artery pulsating. (The number on the pressure gauge when the pulse just disappears is a close approximation of your systolic pressure.) Once the pulse disappears, continue to pump up the pressure about another 30 mm Hg. If, while you are pumping up the pressure, the cuff makes loud crackling sounds, this means that the Velcro lock is slipping. *Stop.* Release the pressure and retighten the cuff.

13b. Pump up the pressure in the cuff with your right hand and at the same time feel the pulse of the brachial artery with the first and second fingers of your left hand. (The number on the pressure gauge when the pulse just disappears is a close approximation of your systolic pressure.) Once the pulse disappears, continue to pump up the pressure about another 30 mm Hg. If, while you are pumping up the pressure, the cuff makes loud crackling sounds, this means that the Velcro lock is slipping. *Stop.* Release the pressure and retighten the cuff.

14a. Transfer the squeeze bulb to your right hand and place the stethoscope head in your left hand.

If you are using electronic equipment or a cuff which has

the stethoscope head permanently attached, Steps 14 and 15 are unnecessary.

14b. Place the stethoscope head in your left hand.

15. Place the stethoscope head gently but firmly over the brachial artery. (You know the location of the artery because you have already identified it with your fingers.) Slightly open the control knob of the release valve at the base of the squeeze bulb. If you have difficulty manipulating the control valve, you can overcome this by purchasing a squeeze bulb which has an automatic release valve. The automatic valve is easier to operate.

16. While carefully watching the pressure gauge, listen for the tapping blood pressure sounds to appear. Note the number on the gauge when the first sound appears. This is the *systolic* blood pressure. Continue listening. The sounds may become softer and they may even disappear. If they do disappear, they will soon return approximately as loud as before. Soon they may again become muffled and soft. Note the number of the gauge when sound can no longer be heard. This is the *diastolic* blood pressure. (Sometimes, the sounds never disappear and can be heard all the way to a pressure reading of zero. This will be discussed under Problems below.)

17. Allow the pressure to drop all the way to zero. Wait a minute or so, and then repeat the blood pressure measurement. Take three measurements. If each blood pressure reading is lower than the one before, continue taking measurements until your blood pressure stabilizes. You may not have been completely rested or completely relaxed when you first started measuring your blood pressure.

18. Never raise the blood pressure in the cuff until you have first allowed the pressure to go to zero; otherwise, falsely high readings can occur.

Problems 1. Difficulty tightening up the blood pressure cuff. The best way to avoid this problem is to buy a cuff that has both a D-ring and a Velcro lock.

2. Difficulty locating the brachial artery. Sometimes the pulsations of the artery are quite soft. It may be necessary to have your physician or a nurse show you how to locate it.

3. Difficulty hearing the sounds. This is *never* the fault of the stethoscope. It is usually due to improper positioning of the stethoscope head above the artery. If you first feel the artery with your fingers, this problem is avoided. If your cuff has the stethoscope head permanently sewn in place or if you are using an electronic device, it is important to be sure that the mark on the cuff is directly over the artery. If you can locate the artery at the junction of the forearm and the upper arm, you can usually assume

that the mark on the cuff will be in line with it on the upper arm. To be absolutely certain that this is the correct location for the mark, you can also feel the artery in the upper arm. It is an inch or two above the elbow on the inner side of the upper arm.

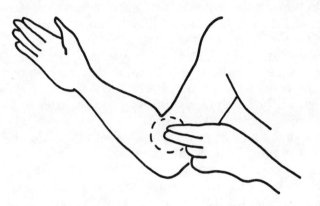

Proper positioning of microphone or permanently attached stethoscope

4. Difficulty catching the very first sound. The best way to solve this problem is first "feel" the first sound and then listen for it. Pump the pressure up until the pulse disappears. Then, instead of placing the stethoscope head over the artery and listening for the first sound, keep your fingers on the artery and allow the pressure to slowly drop. The number on the gauge when you first feel the pulsation of the artery is a close approximation of the systolic blood pressure. Now you know the approximate pressure at which you should hear the first sound. Let the pressure in the cuff drop all the way to zero and start over again. (Remember always to let the pressure go down to zero before again pumping up the cuff.) Now when you listen over the artery with your stethoscope you will be able to anticipate the first sound. It should appear when the pressure on the gauge is about 5 mm Hg higher than the pressure at which you felt the return of the pulse.

If the pressure drops too rapidly you will also have trouble catching the first sound. The release valve must allow the pressure to drop slowly and steadily. It should fall no faster than 2 to 3 mm Hg per second. If you cannot easily adjust the control knob of the valve so that the pressure in the cuff falls slowly and evenly, return the cuff and have it checked. It may need a new release valve.

5. Difficulty deciding when the last sound is heard. This takes practice because you are listening for the *absence* of sound. Here is one way you can concentrate on the disappearance of the sound. Go back to Step 16. When the sound seems to just disappear, instead of allowing the pressure to fall to zero, give the bulb a little squeeze to bring the pressure up a bit. Now the sound

should come back. Since slight changes in the pressure allow the sounds to appear and to disappear, you know that you are close to the diastolic pressure. You now know the approximate reading on the pressure gauge when you should no longer hear the tapping sounds. Repeat the entire blood pressure measurement (starting from zero pressure) and pay particularly close attention when the pressure falls into the range that you now know is close to the diastolic pressure. Once you have developed a little experience in manipulating the squeeze bulb and control valve with your right hand, you should be able to easily raise and lower the pressure so that it is just above the diastolic pressure (sounds present) and just below the diastolic pressure (sounds no longer present).

6. The sounds never disappear. If the heart beats too rapidly (fast pulse) there may be turbulance even though there is no pressure in the cuff to deform the artery. This is often true in children, and it sometimes happens in adults, especially if they are very nervous. If you hear the sounds all the way to a pressure of zero, then you should record the number on the gauge when the sounds go from very clear tapping sounds to muffled soft tapping sounds. This is a reasonable approximation of the diastolic pressure.

Of course, the best solution to this problem is to remedy the cause of the rapid heartbeat. Once a child or an adult becomes accustomed to the procedure, nervousness should lessen and pulse should slow down. Occasionally, a continued rapid pulse is not due to nervousness but rather due to a medical condition. If the pulse seems always to be too rapid, check with your doctor.

Rarely, the tapping sounds may persist because the stethoscope head is pressed too firmly over the artery. The stethoscope head should be held securely but gently over the artery.

7. Successive blood pressure readings vary widely from each other. This will occur only with the electronic devices, and it means that the battery is worn down. Replace the battery.

8. Lots of extra noises in addition to the tapping sounds. This indicates that you are moving your right arm too much. The muscle of the right arm must remain still and relaxed.

The instructions provided above may differ from those which accompany your blood pressure kit. Most of the diagrams provided in kits, for example, show blood pressure measured with the cuff located on the left arm instead of the right. True, it is easier to perform one-handed steps using the right hand instead of the left but, as noted earlier, this will not provide the most accurate reading in the majority of cases. If the instructions in your kit show a left-hand reading or differ in other ways from those provided in the step-by-step procedure in the chapter, discuss with your doctor how to proceed.

16

THE PRUDENT DIET

If you are like most people, when you hear the word "diet," you probably think of "going hungry." What an unpleasant thought! Fortunately, this is not what doctors mean when they recommend the "prudent diet." The prudent diet is not a method of weight loss, so you will not be burdened with following diet charts. It is a style of eating that has been proven to help prevent heart disease. You will be happy to learn that you can follow the prudent diet and never feel hungry. The diet is "prudent" because it is now well known that those who follow it decrease their risk of suffering a heart attack or experiencing some other form of serious heart disease. If you want to improve your chances of living a long and healthy life, it is wise to follow the "prudent diet"!

A LOOK AT THE PAST

Before 1900, heart attacks were extremely rare. Medical scientists had already determined that the underlying cause of heart attacks was atherosclerosis (hardening of the arteries due to fat and cholesterol buildups within the arterial walls). They even had an idea that the development of atherosclerosis had something to do with the way people ate, but the problem affected so few people that very little research was devoted to this subject. Then, over the next forty years, heart disease—and especially heart attacks—increased at an alarming rate in many areas of the world. Not only was there much more heart disease, but it was affecting people at an incredibly early age. Men were dying of heart attacks while still in their thirties, something which was previously unknown. Why was this happening, and why was death due to heart attack a frequent occurrence in some parts of the world and a rare event in others? Unfortunately, World War II came along and diverted all the money and energy that might otherwise have been spent finding the answers to these questions. It was only in 1945 that scientists finally had the opportunity to turn their attention to these critical issues.

Early in the investigations, it became clear that heart attacks occurred mainly in those areas of the world where people enjoyed a high standard of living. There were still many countries where heart attacks were almost unheard of. This was a major clue that perhaps lifestyle had something to do with the early onset of heart disease. If this was true, then it was also true that lifestyle played an important role in producing early atherosclerosis, because it was already known that heart attacks and atherosclerosis go together.

To find out why heart attacks and heart disease had become so common, medical scientists decided upon three types of experiments. In one type, they compared people who lived in different parts of the world. What made people who lived in an area where there was a low rate of heart attack different from people who lived in an area where heart attack had become so common? In another, so-called longitudinal type of experiment, scientists studied a large number of people all living in the same community. As time went on, it could be anticipated that some would develop heart disease and some would not. By examining everyone at regular intervals over a number of years, perhaps the scientists would be able to identify something that distinguished those who eventually suffered heart attacks from those who did not. Finally, scientists began feeding experimental diets to animals to see whether certain kinds of food could produce atherosclerosis. There was already strong reason to believe that diet played a role in causing atherosclerosis, because as early as 1909 German scientists had demonstrated that diets very high in cholesterol produced atherosclerosis in experimental animals.

Within ten years, all three types of experiments produced evidence which strongly suggested that lifestyle did indeed play a major role in the development of atherosclerosis. For example, it became clear that atherosclerosis (and therefore heart diseases) does in fact mainly affect individuals who enjoy a high standard of living. The studies also revealed that, on the average, those who live in comparatively wealthy countries have much higher levels of blood cholesterol and blood fats than those who live in less fortunate areas of the world. Lifestyle is strongly implicated in producing this difference, because in countries where heart attacks are prevalent, blood cholesterol and blood fats are high, while in countries where heart attacks are rare, blood cholesterol and blood fat levels are low. In those countries where heart attacks are prevalent, the population consumes large quantities of meat, eggs, milk fats, and refined sugar. In those countries where heart attacks are rare, meat is scarce, and the people eat mainly fish, vegetables, and grains. The evidence strongly suggests that the way people eat has a major role in producing atherosclerosis by raising the level of blood cholesterol and blood fats.

The same conclusions came out of the longitudinal studies,

in which a large number of people who all live in the same community were examined repeatedly over a long period of years. It soon became clear that those individuals who were destined to develop heart disease had one or more features which made them different from those who remained free of heart disease. Cigarette smokers have more heart attacks than nonsmokers. Individuals who have high blood pressure have more heart attacks than those whose blood pressure remains normal. Obese individuals who have high blood cholesterol and high blood fat levels have more heart attacks than those whose blood cholesterol and blood fat levels remain low. Thus cigarette smoking, high blood pressure, obesity, high blood cholesterol, and high blood fats were identified as "risk factors" for the development of heart disease. All of these risk factors except high blood pressure are related to lifestyle.

While these studies were going on, experiments with laboratory animals confirmed the early German observation that a high-cholesterol diet could induce atherosclerosis. An important finding of these experiments was that atherosclerosis could also be produced by feeding animals diets that were high in fat—but not just *any* kind of fat. Only the kind of fat known as *saturated fat* produced atherosclerosis, and this kind of fat is found mainly in meat and milk products. This was additional evidence that lifestyle is indeed of primary importance to the development of atherosclerosis.

By 1957 most nutritionists and many physicians were convinced that the ingestion of a diet high in cholesterol and saturated fats was a major contributor to the epidemic of heart attacks and other forms of heart diseases in certain nations. It was already known that the arteries which supplied blood to the heart, the *coronary arteries*, become narrowed and clogged because of the buildup of abnormal chemical deposits within their walls (atherosclerosis) and that these abnormal deposits consist mainly of cholesterol and fats. Scientists now knew that diets high in cholesterol and saturated fats predisposed the individual to atherosclerosis. It was only logical to assume that "coronary heart disease," the big killer, was related to a high-cholesterol and high-fat diet, and that "coronary mortality" could be reduced if people were willing to change their eating habits. The time had come to put this idea to the test.

In 1957 the New York City Health Department recommended what has since become known as the "prudent diet." The major features of this diet are a reduction in cholesterol, saturated fats, and refined sugar, and an increase in what is known as *unsaturated fat*. The diet was tested over a ten-year period, and by 1967 it had become obvious that the diet worked. Men who followed the diet experienced *less than one-half* as many heart attacks as those who continued to follow the "normal" American diet. Since that time, this experiment has been tested in other populations, and the results have been the same. It is clear that *individuals who are willing to decrease the amount of cholesterol, saturated fats, and refined sugar that they eat can decrease their risk of heart attack and other forms of heart disease.*

Americans must be doing something right, because since 1968 the death rate from coronary heart disease has been on the decline even though the number of people reaching an old age has increased.

In the last ten years Americans have decreased their consumption of whole milk and cream by 20 percent, their consumption of butter by 35 percent, and their consumption of eggs by 10 percent. Americans are now cooking with less lard (a saturated fat), and using 44 percent more vegetable oils (unsaturated fats), eating leaner meats, and consuming more poultry and fish. Although the control of high blood pressure, the curtailment of cigarette smoking, the correction of obesity, the better availability of medical care, and the participation in more regular physical exercise also play a role, there is little doubt that the alteration in the "American way of eating" has been a major contributor to the decline in coronary mortality.

While the coronary death rate is on the decline in America, it is on the rise in many other countries. Most medical scientists believe that this rise in deaths due to heart disease is related to a shift to "eating, American style" (foods high in cholesterol, saturated fats, and refined sugar) as the standard of living improves. The increasing death rate due to coronary heart disease in countries with an improved standard of living is further evidence that lifestyle is an important contributor to the development of atherosclerosis.

There is now convincing evidence that a change in the way that you eat can lower the level of your blood cholesterol and blood fats, and that this can, in turn, slow down the development of atherosclerosis. There is little doubt that the prudent diet is a heart saver, and it is strongly recommended, in addition to keeping your blood pressure under control, maintaining a normal weight, stopping cigarette smoking, and engaging in regular physical exercise, that you also follow the dietary recommendations of the prudent diet.

The prudent diet is low in cholesterol and low in saturated fats. Unsaturated fats do not raise the cholesterol level, and in the prudent diet the amount of saturated fats (animal fats) is reduced and replaced with unsaturated fats (vegetable and fish oils). Also, the amount of refined sugar, which has been shown to raise the level of blood fats (triglycerides), is reduced and replaced with complex sugars (carbohydrates and starches) which naturally occur in vegetables, fruits, grains, breads, and legumes.

REDUCE YOUR INTAKE OF FOOD RICH IN CHOLESTEROL

Your body utilizes the chemical *cholesterol* as a building block to synthesize other chemicals which are important to your metabolism. Many hormones, for example, are synthesized from cholesterol. Cholesterol is found only in foods of animal origin, and it is present in large amounts in only a few foods. For this reason, it is relatively easy to cut down on cholesterol consumption. All that is required is that you either give up or significantly cut down on egg yolks, meats (especially organ meats), and whole milk and whole milk products.

Since pure vegetarians eat no food of animal origin at all, you might wonder how they get cholesterol. Actually, if you eat no cholesterol, your body will manufacture cholesterol out of other chemicals. Thus, it is normal to have a certain amount of cholesterol in your bloodstream at all times even if you do not eat any foods which contain it. Your body will regulate its cholesterol level so that your metabolism remains normal whether or not you eat cholesterol-containing foods.

The prudent diet recommends that you reduce your cholesterol consumption to no more than 300 milligrams (mg) per day. One egg yolk contains about 245 mg of cholesterol (there is no cholesterol in egg white), so you can see that eggs have to be almost entirely eliminated from your diet. Most physicians now recommend no more than two eggs per week, and certainly four per week should be the upper limit. Four ounces of raw liver (three ounces cooked) provides about 497 mg of cholesterol. This exceeds the daily recommended allowance, and you will have to limit liver and the other organ meats to certainly no more than once every two weeks.

Most lean meat, poultry, fish, and shellfish provide about 60 to 110 mg of cholesterol per four-ounce raw serving (three ounces cooked). The fattier the meat or fish, the higher in cholesterol content, so lean is better than fatty. Poultry skin is another high-cholesterol food so poultry should be eaten without the skin. Shrimp is an exception among the shellfish. Shrimp has about three times the cholesterol content of the other shellfish and should be limited. Whole milk, butter, cheese, and all other products made from whole milk provide cholesterol, and the higher the milk fat content, the higher the content of cholesterol. Since skim milk is essentially fat free, it is also essentially free of cholesterol.

A cup of whole milk provides about 32 mg of cholesterol, but a cup of skim milk provides only 5 mg.

Cheeses are a concentrated form of milk fat, and an ounce of most cheeses (one slice) provides about 30 mg of cholesterol. It is now possible to buy cheese made from partially skimmed milk (for example, mozzarella and skim milk cottage cheese), and these cheeses contain only about 15 mg of cholesterol per ounce. Ice cream is a rich source of milk fat and therefore a reasonably rich source of cholesterol. Regular ice cream contains 10 percent milk fat, and one cup provides about 50 mg of cholesterol.

In order to keep within the recommended daily allowance of 300 mg of cholesterol, you will have to do more than strictly limit the quantity of eggs and organ meats that you consume. You will have to switch to skim milk and skim milk products and cut down on those foods which are high in milk fats (butter, cream, cheese, and ice cream). You will also have to reduce your consumption of highly fatty meats and emphasize lean cuts of meat, poultry without skin, fish, and seafood. (You will have to do this anyway, because, as you will soon learn, it is necessary to limit the major sources of *animal fat* in order to reduce your consumption of saturated fats.) Remember that foods of plant origin contain *no* cholesterol, and all vegetables, legumes, grains, fruits, and vegetable oils (except coconut oil and cocoa butter) can be eaten freely.

Most bakery products and desserts do contain some cholesterol because usually either egg yolk, whole milk, or cheese is added.

The following table will show you the cholesterol content of many of the common food items:

CHOLESTEROL CONTENT OF SOME COMMON FOOD ITEMS

TYPE OF FOOD	SERVING SIZE	APPROXIMATE CHOLESTEROL CONTENT
MEAT (cooked)		
lean beef	3 oz.	107 mg
beef liver	3 oz.	370 mg
"all beef" hot dog	2 oz. (1 hot dog)	50 mg
lamb	3 oz.	112 mg
pork, ham	3 oz.	100 mg
bacon	2 slices	15 mg
pork sausages	3 oz.	80 mg
veal	3 oz.	115 mg

TYPE OF FOOD	SERVING SIZE	APPROXIMATE CHOLESTEROL CONTENT
FISH (cooked)		
haddock	3 oz.	68 mg
halibut	3 oz.	57 mg
herring	3 oz.	96 mg
mackerel	3 oz.	108 mg
salmon	3 oz.	53 mg
trout	3 oz.	62 mg
tuna	3 oz.	62 mg
SHELLFISH (cooked)		
clams	3 oz.	40 mg
oysters	3 oz.	57 mg
scallops	3 oz.	45 mg
shrimp	3 oz.	170 mg
POULTRY (cooked)		
chicken (light meat with skin)	3 oz.	65 mg
turkey (light meat with skin)	3 oz.	68 mg
egg yolk	1 egg	245 mg
egg white	any amount	0 mg
MILK PRODUCTS		
whole milk	8 oz. (1 cup)	32 mg
skim milk	8 oz. (1 cup)	5 mg
butter	½ oz. (1 Tbsp.)	30 mg
cheeses:		
uncreamed cottage cheese	8 oz. (1 cup)	16 mg
creamed cottage cheese	8 oz. (1 cup)	45 mg
American	1 oz.	30 mg
Edam	1 oz.	30 mg
farmers	1 oz.	6 mg
mozzarella (part-skim)	1 oz.	18 mg

TYPE OF FOOD	SERVING SIZE	APPROXIMATE CHOLESTEROL CONTENT
cheeses (continued):		
Muenster	1 oz.	25 mg
Parmesan	1 oz.	25 mg
Provolone	1 oz.	27 mg
ricotta	1 oz.	14 mg
Swiss	1 oz.	28 mg
DESSERTS		
chocolate cake	1/16 of 9-inch cake	32 mg
angel food cake	any amount	0 mg
baked custard	1 cup	275 mg
regular ice cream (10% fat)	1 cup	50 mg
sherbet	any amount	0 mg
COOKING OILS		
lard	½ oz. (1 Tbsp.)	12 mg
margarine	any amount	0 mg
vegetable oils	any amount	0 mg

REDUCE YOUR INTAKE OF FOOD RICH IN SATURATED FATS

There are two types of fats: saturated and unsaturated. All *animal* food sources, except fish, contain saturated fats. Fish is an excellent source of unsaturated fats. All *vegetable* food sources are unsaturated except coconut oil and chocolate (cocoa butter). It is easy to tell a saturated fat from an unsaturated fat: saturated fats are firm at room temperature and unsaturated fats are liquid at room temperature.

There are also two types of unsaturated fats: monounsaturated and polyunsaturated. Polyunsaturated fats are the most desirable type of the two because polyunsaturated fats have somewhat of a cholesterol-lowering effect. Monounsaturated fats are considered "neutral". That is, monounsaturated fats neither raise nor lower your blood cholesterol. In short:

Saturated fats raise blood cholesterol and are undesirable.

Polyunsaturated fats have a cholesterol-lowering effect and are desirable.

Monounsaturated fats neither raise nor lower cholesterol; they are neutral.

Generally, when you read or hear of "unsaturated fats," this usually refers to fats of the polyunsaturated variety.

Hydrogenation

It is possible to convert an unsaturated fat into a saturated fat, and it is important that you understand this, because food manufacturers frequently make such a conversion in order to enhance a food product's marketability. The classic example of this is margarine. Think about corn oil margarine for a moment. Corn oil (like all other vegetable oils except coconut oil) is an unsaturated fat, yet corn oil margarine is firm at room temperature. How can that be? The answer is simply that the manufacturer has chemically converted some of the desirable naturally unsaturated corn oil into a less desirable saturated form by a chemical process called *hydrogenation*. Why did the manufacturer do this? So that the margarine would have a firm consistency. If it didn't, would you want to buy it?

All vegetable oils except coconut oil are desirable as long as they are not hydrogenated. Most baked goods, snack foods, candies, and other confections have "partially hydrogentated vegetable oils" added. To the extent possible, you should try to buy products that are made with vegetable oils, but not partially hydrogenated oils. You should also try to avoid buying products that contain coconut oil. If you do any cooking with fats or oils, always use a liquid vegetable oil.

Foods Rich in Saturated Fats

Meat and Poultry All animal sources of protein except fish and shellfish contain mainly saturated fat. Consequently, when you purchase meat or poultry, it is desirable to purchase cuts that are *low in fat*. All poultry except duck and goose is reasonably low in fat, so poultry presents little problem. Lean beef, lamb, pork, and veal all have about the same fat content, but the fat in veal is less saturated than the others and therefore is more desirable. Variety meats such as hot dogs, sausages, cold cuts, and luncheon meats are high in saturated fat, because the fatty scraps of the meat are used in their preparation. Do not let labels fool you. An "all beef" hot dog does not mean a "low-fat" hot dog. "All beef" means only that the fatty meat used to stuff the hot dog comes from a beef source. All meat and poultry should be kept to about four-ounce (raw) portions and should be broiled or baked. (Before cooking, all the visible fat should be removed.) Broiling and baking help to eliminate fat, but frying does not. Fast food meat items tend to be high in fat and should be avoided.

Milk and Milk Products Whole milk and whole milk products are a major source of saturated fats. This means that butter, cream, cheeses, and ice cream are high in saturated fats. Skim milk, however, is low in fat (99 percent fat free) and products made from skim milk are also low in fat. It is now possible to purchase cheeses made from skim milk (for example, mozzarella, dry cottage cheese, and dry ricotta cheese) and fat-free ice creams, ices, and sherbets are also available. You should eliminate whole milk, butter, and cream from your diet, limit cheeses, and purchase skim milk products whenever possible.

Cooking Fats and Oils Lard is pure animal fat and should be avoided. Butter and coconut oil are also rich sources of saturated fats. Margarine and hydrogenated shortenings should have more of the fat as unsaturated than saturated. The label of a margarine or hydrogenated shortening product will look something like this:

MARGARINE—NUTRITION INFORMATION PER SERVING

Serving size ....1 Tbsp. (14 grams)
Servings per 1 lb. container 32
Calories 100
Protein 0
Carbohydrate 0
Fat ....11 grams
    Polyunsaturated ....5 grams
    Saturated ....2 grams
Cholesterol 0

The important information is given below the listing "Fat." You know that the total amount of fat is 11 grams. Of this, 5 grams are polyunsaturated and 2 grams are saturated. Thus, there are more polyunsaturated fats present than saturated fats. Clearly 4 grams of fat are missing from the total. Do not be concerned. This means that 4 grams of fat are the monounsaturated variety, so they don't particularly have any health benefit but on the other hand they aren't harmful to you either. When you purchase margarine and hydrogenated vegetable shortenings, compare labels and buy the product which has the most polyunsaturated and the least saturated fats.

Eggs The fat in egg yolks is saturated. Egg white does not contain fat.

Bakery Products, Snack Foods, Candies, and Confections Most bakery products, snack foods, candies, and other confections contain coconut oil (a saturated fat) as well as partially hydrogenated vegetable oils. Chocolate (cocoa butter) is also a saturated fat, and a chocolate candy usually contains not only the saturated fat from the chocolate, but also saturated fat from coconut oil, hydrogenated vegetable oils, and whole milk. Many food manufacturers are beginning to take notice of the consumer demand for products prepared with unsaturated oils. You should now be able to purchase chips and crackers made, for example, with soy oil, corn oil, or some other pure vegetable oil.

Foods Rich in Unsaturated Fats (Desirable)
This is an easy group to remember. All vegetables and vegetable oils except coconut oil and chocolate (cocoa butter) are rich in unsaturated fats (monounsaturated and polyunsaturated). Such foods as seeds, nuts, grains, cereals, and legumes fall into this classification. Fish is also an excellent source of unsaturated fats (mainly polyunsaturated). The best way to increase your intake of polyunsaturated fats is to use only vegetable oils (often called salad oils) for cooking and to eat more fish. Some vegetable oils are more polyunsaturated than others. The most desirable vegetable oils are corn oil, cottonseed oil, soybean oil, peanut oil, and safflower oil. Remember: No food of vegetable origin contains cholesterol.

The following table summarizes the types of fat contained in various foods. Remember, saturated fats are undesirable, and polyunsaturated fats are desirable.

FOODS WHICH PREDOMINATELY CONTAIN SATURATED FATS	FOODS WHICH PREDOMINATELY CONTAIN UNSATURATED (POLYUNSATURATED) FATS
Bakery products	Fish
Butter	Margarine
Cheese	Nuts
Cream	Vegetable oils:
Chocolate	corn oil
Coconut and coconut oil	cottonseed oil
Eggs	peanut oil
Ice Cream	safflower oil
Whole milk	soybean oil
Lard	
Meat	

You may have noticed that olive oil is not listed in the above table. Olive oil contains predominately monounsaturated fats, which are neutral.

WHAT ABOUT SUGAR?

There is still some controversy about how important it is for you
to limit the amount of refined sugar that you eat. The complex sugars (carbohydrates, starches) found in rice, wheat, grains, cereals,
fruits, legumes, vegetables, and bread need not be limited unless
you have a specific abnormality of your metabolism called *Type IV
hyperlipidemia* (which will be discussed later). Since fewer than
one in twenty individuals have this condition, it is unlikely that
you have any reason to limit the amount of complex sugars that
you eat unless you need to lose weight. However, there is evidence
which suggests that the continued ingestion of high amounts of *refined sugar* (cane sugar, brown sugar, dextrose, sucrose, glucose,
fructose) can raise the level of blood fats (triglycerides) and indi-
rectly raise the blood cholesterol level. Since the ingestion of refined sugar is, in any event, the major cause of dental caries (cav-
ities), and since there is evidence suggesting that the continued
high intake of refined sugar contributes to the development of
early atherosclerosis, it seems wise to recommend that you reduce
your daily intake.

        The major sources of refined sugar in your diet are soft
drink beverages, the added sugar in coffee and tea, and the sugar
in bakery products, cereals, and candies. By simply omitting soft
drinks, switching to a cereal with no added sugar, and not adding
sugar to your coffee, tea, and cereal, you will probably reduce your
daily intake of refined sugar to a safe level. Instead of adding sugar
to your cereal, add a naturally sweet fruit such as a banana. Instead of adding sugar to tea or coffee, add honey. (Although fructose is now being promoted as the new miracle sweetener, evidence suggests that fructose is an even more potent elevator of
blood fats than is cane sugar or sucrose.

WHAT ABOUT ALCOHOL?

Physicians and nutritionists agree that a moderate alcohol intake
is not harmful. The difficulty is in deciding what "moderate"
means. The amount of alcohol that you can safely drink in a day
continues to be a source of controversy. At one time, it was
thought that the equivalent of six to eight ounces of 100 proof
whiskey was safe, but now this is thought to be too high. The most
recent evidence suggests you should keep your daily alcohol consumption to about the equivalent of two ounces of 100 proof
whiskey.

WHAT ABOUT CALORIES?

Up to this point in the discussion of the prudent diet, no mention
has been made of the need to restrict the total number of calories

that you eat in a day. *This description of the prudent diet is intended for individuals who are NOT overweight!* If you are overweight, you should still follow the prudent diet, but you should also cut down on the total amount of food that you eat each day until you have achieved a desirable weight. Obesity is associated with high blood fat and cholesterol levels, and weight reduction is extremely important if you wish to reduce the risk of developing atherosclerosis. If you are overweight, it may be very difficult for you to achieve a reduction in your cholesterol and blood fat levels if you follow the prudent diet but remain obese.

What does it mean to have a desirable weight? It means to have a weight which studies have demonstrated are *not* associated with premature death. The best information on desirable weights comes from life insurance companies, because life insurance companies make their money by predicting how long you will live. These companies know that individuals who are overweight are bad insurance risks, because overweight individuals have a higher probability of dying prematurely than individuals who maintain a normal weight. Recently, the insurance companies changed their tables of desirable weights, making them about ten pounds lower than the old tables. The following table will help you to determine your desirable weight.

If you are more than about 10 percent over the weight listed for your age in these tables, then it is suggested that you not only follow the prudent diet but also go on a weight reduction program. What you will want to find is a responsible program which emphasizes the food practices of the prudent diet. If you feel you can most successfully lose weight by joining a group program, you are encouraged to join a *responsible* program such as Weight Watchers. Avoid faddist diets. Nutritionally, they are undesirable, and, in any event, they seldom lead to a true weight loss. Most faddist diets do no more than produce an initial fluid loss. Very few who follow them ever achieve a permanent weight loss.

WHAT ABOUT FIBER?

Foods of vegetable origin are high in fiber. There is reason to believe that the increased intake of vegetable fiber helps to lower blood cholesterol. The degree of effect may be small, but it is probably real. Vegetable fiber is thought to bind the cholesterol that is released as food is digested in your intestine and, in this way, prevent some of the released cholesterol from being absorbed into your bloodstream. Since the prudent diet encourages the reduction of animal foods and an increase in vegetable foods, you will naturally achieve whatever benefit there is from a high-fiber diet. At one time physicians believed that vegetable fiber intake should be

...

HEALTHIEST WEIGHT FOR MEN AND WOMEN

Assumes you are wearing indoor clothing without shoes.

Age:	15-16	17-19	20-24	25-29	30-39	40-49	50-59	60-69
Height								
4' 8"	91	93	95	99	102	106	109	111
4' 9"	95	97	99	101	104	109	112	114
4'10"	98	100	101	103	106	111	114	117
4'11"	101	104	104	107	109	114	117	120
5' 0"	105	107	108	110	112	116	120	122
5' 1"	109	111	112	113	115	120	123	126
	101	115	123	126	128	128	127	126
5' 2"	112	113	114	116	118	122	127	129
	105	117	124	127	129	130	131	130
5' 3"	115	116	117	119	121	125	130	132
	109	119	126	129	132	134	135	134
5' 4"	118	119	120	121	123	129	133	135
	114	123	129	132	136	139	140	138
5' 5"	122	122	123	124	127	132	137	139
	120	127	133	136	140	142	143	142
5' 6"	125	126	127	128	131	135	140	142
	124	131	138	140	144	147	148	147
5' 7"	128	130	131	132	135	139	143	145
	129	135	141	145	149	150	151	150
5' 8"	131	133	134	135	138	142	146	147
	133	140	147	150	153	155	156	155
5' 9"	134	135	139	140	143	146	149	150
	138	144	150	154	157	158	159	158
5'10"	137	139	142	143	148	151	154	155
	143	148	154	158	161	163	164	163
5'11"	146	151	158	163	166	167	168	167
6' 0"	151	156	163	167	171	173	174	172
6' 1"	156	161	168	172	176	177	178	176
6' 2"	160	167	174	177	181	183	184	181
6' 3"	166	171	178	182	185	187	188	186

Developed by Pacific Mutual Life Insurance Company from a study by the Association of Life Insurance Medical Directors and the Society of Actuaries.

reduced among sufferers trom such intestinal disorders as diverti-
culitis, colitis, irritable bowel, spastic bowel, and ulcer disease.
This is now known to be false. In fact, a high-fiber diet is helpful
because it prevents constipation. There is no medical condition
that is made worse by a diet that has an increased quantity of vegetable fiber and such a diet should be encouraged.

WHAT ABOUT VEGETARIANISM?

True vegetarians are people who do not eat meat, fish, poultry, or
any animal products, such as eggs, milk, or cheese. True vegetarians have very low levels of blood cholesterol and fats, and cultures
that practice true vegetarianism tend to have low rates of heart
disease. True vegetarianism is compatible with good health, but it
does require a real knowledge of the vegetable sources of protein
if protein deficiency is to be avoided.

Proteins are complex molecules which perform a number of
important roles. For example: Much of the structural framework
of the body is made up of protein; proteins are vital to every aspect
of our metabolism, and without them, it is impossible to obtain
energy from the food we eat or to synthesize vital chemicals; and
the antibodies which are essential to combat infection are proteins.

The large protein molecules are made up of smaller molecules called amino acids. Amino acids can be considered to be the
building blocks from which all proteins are constructed. There are
many amino acids. Some we are able to manufacture ourselves;
others must be obtained from our food. Those amino acids that we
cannot synthesize are called *essential amino acids*, because it is essential that we obtain them from our food. We obtain amino acids
from plant and animal protein sources. When plant and animal
protein is eaten, our digestive process separates the proteins into
their component amino acids. The amino acids are taken into the
body, and we then use them to form new proteins. If a particular
food is able to provide us with *all* the essential amino acids we require, it is called a *complete protein food*—or just a *complete protein*. Meat and fish are complete proteins. Some food sources have
some but not all of the essential amino acids. These food sources
are called *incomplete proteins*. Most vegetable sources of protein
are incomplete, because they tend to be lacking in one or more of
the required amino acids. It is also possible for a food to have all
of the essential amino acids and still be an inadequate protein
source, because one or more of the essential amino acids may be
present in such small quantities it is not possible to eat enough of
the food to obtain an adequate supply of the amino acid. Not only
must we eat foods which supply all of the essential amino acids,

but we must also eat foods which provide us with an adequate quantity of each. For this reason, vegetarians must eat a mixture of plant proteins. In this way, an amino acid which may be absent or only present in low amounts in one plant protein source can be supplemented by another plant protein source which has an abundant supply of that amino acid. The best sources of vegetable protein are grains, cereals, and legumes. The only complete plant protein source is the soybean. For the true vegetarian to obtain all the required amino acids, a mixture of grains, cereals, and legumes is required, and emphasis on the soybean is preferable. The true vegetarian also needs a Vitamin B_{12} supplement, because Vitamin B_{12} comes mainly from meat and eggs.

Many people who follow a vegetarian practice are not true vegetarians. They may eat fish, poultry, eggs, or dairy products (milk and cheeses). Those who supplement the vegetarian diet with fish or poultry and skim milk are essentially following the prudent diet. Those who supplement the vegetarian diet with large amounts of eggs or whole milk products do not receive the beneficial effects of a vegetarian practice, because eggs are high in cholesterol, and whole milk products are high both in saturated fats and cholesterol.

WHAT ABOUT VITAMINS?

The prudent diet is a balanced diet, and there is probably no urgent reason to take a multivitamin. However, meat is a good source of many mineral elements (especially iron) and since the prudent diet does cut down meat intake, the addition of a multivitamin supplement with iron and other minerals may be of some value. Although excessive amounts of vitamins can prove harmful (especially if large amounts of the fat-soluble vitamins are taken), there is no harm in taking one or two multivitamin supplements with minerals daily, and it may even be beneficial.

WHAT ABOUT EXERCISE?

The best information suggests that regular physical exercise does not protect against the development of early atherosclerosis if obesity and blood pressure are not also controlled and if a diet similar to the prudent diet is not followed. Probably much of the beneficial effect of regular exercise comes from the attention that those who exercise also pay to diet, cigarette smoking, blood pressure, and weight. One of the best ways to control your weight is to participate regularly in an exercise program, and regular exercise is also of some help in bringing a mild elevation of blood pressure down to normal. You are strongly encouraged to engage in a program of regular physical exercises, but do not assume that exercise is a substitute for the prudent diet—it is not.

HYPERLIPIDEMIA

Should your doctor measure your blood cholesterol and blood fat levels? Cessation of cigarette smoking, control of blood pressure, correction of obesity, and acceptance of the prudent diet will provide maximum protection against the development of early heart disease for at least 95 out of every 100 people. About 5 percent or less will need to follow a diet slightly different from the prudent diet. These individuals suffer from one of the inherited deficiencies of fat metabolism called *hyperlipidemia*.

There are five types of hyperlipidemia, but only two are common enough to be worth mentioning: Type II and Type IV. Individuals with Type II hyperlipidemia have very high cholesterol levels that cannot be brought completely under control by the prudent diet alone. Individuals who have this form of abnormal metabolism must take *extra* amounts of polyunsaturated fats. More than 95 out of 100 people will *not* benefit from extra amounts of polyunsaturated fats, so you should go to the trouble of eating more only if you have Type II hyperlipidemia. Individuals with Type IV hyperlipidemia have abnormally high levels of blood fats (triglycerides), and the blood fat level will not be brought completely under control by the prudent diet. These individuals must also restrict their intake of carbohydrates and starches. Their metabolisms tend to be very sensitive to alcohol, and Type IV individuals must severely limit their intake of alcohol as well.

If your doctor has any reason to suspect that you might be one of the relatively rare individuals who has an abnormal fat metabolism, then your cholesterol and triglyceride level should be measured. Who is likely to have such a condition? Since these conditions are inherited, family history becomes important. If members of your immediate family have developed heart disease at an early age, then you should be checked. If *you* have developed heart disease at an early age, this is another reason to check. Often individuals with abnormalities of their fat metabolism develop telltale signs on their skin. If you or members of your family have deposits in the skin about the eyes or in the palms of the hands, this is another good reason to have your blood cholesterol and blood triglyceride level measured.

The recent ingestion of a meal does not affect the measurement of blood cholesterol, but it is impossible to accurately measure your blood triglyceride level if you have eaten within 12 hours of the blood test. Furthermore, your last meal before the test should not be excessively fatty, and alcohol should be limited to only a small amount. The measurement of blood triglycerides is not as simple as the measurement of blood cholesterol, because many disease conditions and a few medications will cause the level of blood triglycerides to rise. Remember, the purpose of the test is to determine whether you are one of the unusual people who have an *inherited* abnormality of your fat metabolism. Since certain disease states and medicines can also cause fat metabolism to be abnormal, your doctor must be certain that you do not have one of these medical conditions before labeling you as having an inherited condition. Here are the major conditions which raise the blood triglyceride level: any acute stress such as a heart attack, serious infection, or operation; diabetes mellitus; and underactive thyroid; diseases of the liver, pancreas, or kidney; alcoholism. The only major medications which raise the blood triglyceride level are the oral contraceptive pill and diuretics, but the health significance of this is not known.

WHAT SHOULD YOUR DOCTOR DO?

Your doctor should definitely not allow you to smoke cigarettes. Cigarette smoking is a major risk factor in the development of heart disease, and it makes no sense to go to the trouble of changing your eating style if you are going to continue to smoke cigarettes.

Your doctor should definitely advise you to lose weight if you are overweight, and your doctor should help you undertake a responsible weight reduction program that incorporates the features of the prudent diet.

Your doctor should definitely bring your blood pressure down to normal levels if it is elevated. High blood pressure is a major risk factor in the development of heart disease, and most of the benefits of the prudent diet will be lost if your blood pressure is not also controlled. Salt restriction and weight reduction may be all that is required. If these two measures do not work, then medication is a must.

If there is reason to believe that you may have an abnormality of fat metabolism, then your doctor should check your cholesterol and triglyceride levels.

WHAT ABOUT YOUR CHILDREN?

The prudent diet is good for you, and it is even better for your children. The earlier this protective lifestyle is initiated, the better. Most physicians now suggest that you begin the prudent diet when your child is about two years of age. If you are found to have one of the unusual abnormalities of fat metabolism discussed above, then it becomes extremely important that your children also be tested. These conditions are inherited, and if you have one, your child might also be affected.

WHAT WILL THE FUTURE BRING?

Meat, whole milk, whole milk products, and eggs are all sources of both saturated fats and cholesterol. For now, it is necessary for you to reduce your intake of these foods if you wish to retard the development of atherosclerosis. This might not be true in the future. Recent experiments have demonstrated that it is possible to produce meat and milk which have a higher proportion of the desirable unsaturated fats and to produce eggs which are lower in cholesterol. To achieve these desirable results, the animals must be fed special-formula diets. Presently, the cost is too high to produce these altered food products in large enough amounts to be meaningful. Perhaps this will change at a future date.

Of more immediate interest are the new meat and egg substitutes. These food items are produced from vegetable proteins (mainly soybean) and contain no cholesterol and decreased amounts of saturated fats. As food manufacturers gain experience, they are able to produce food items which retain much of the flavor and texture of the foods we have become accustomed to eating. Many such products are now available, and it can be anticipated that many more will become available in the future. As the price of meat and fish continues to rise, it is likely that these new products will be desirable not only because of their health benefit, but also because they will provide a less expensive source of protein.

SUMMARY OF THE PRUDENT DIET

The prudent diet is a way of eating which eliminates little but which modifies much. It is designed to lessen your intake of cholesterol, saturated fats, and refined sugar. Starches and carbohydrates are not restricted, and unsaturated fats are substituted for the saturated ones. The following guidelines will help you to learn this new style of eating:

1. Reduce your intake of cholesterol by limiting egg yolks to two (and certainly no more than four) per week, by eating no more than four ounces (raw) of meat, poultry, or seafood per day, by eliminating whole milk and whole milk products and substituting skim milk and skim milk products in their place, and by limiting cheese.

2. Reduce your intake of saturated fats by eating no more than four ounces (raw) of meat or poultry per day, by avoiding

fatty meats almost completely, by trimming off all visible fat prior to cooking, and by baking and broiling and never frying.

3. Replace saturated fats with unsaturated fats, cook only with vegetable oils (except coconut oil), and use margarines high in polyunsaturated fats in place of lard or butter. Whenever possible, purchase bakery and snack products cooked with unsaturated vegetable oils rather than with coconut oil and partially hydrogenated vegetable oils.

4. Reduce the amount of refined sugar that you eat by limiting soft drink beverages, cereals with added sugar, and tea and coffee sweetened with sugar.

5. Limit alcohol to the equivalent of about two ounces of 100 proof whiskey per day.

May you enjoy healthful and pleasurable meals the "prudent" way!

17

IT'S UP TO YOU

You now know just about everything that there is to know about high blood pressure and related health issues. You know what blood pressure means, how it is accurately (and not so accurately) measured, when it is too high, and the nature of the careful evaluation that must be performed before any form of treatment is recommended. You know the three basic mechanisms by which medicines regulate blood pressure, and you know the logical sequence in which medicines should be administered. If your doctor prescribes a high blood pressure medication, you are now able not only to make certain that its dosage conforms to the recommended range, but also to ensure that it does not adversely interact with any other medicine you may require, that you experience no untoward side effects, and that special precautions are taken if you are pregnant or nursing or if you have an important medical condition in addition to high blood pressure. Should you be one of those unusual individuals whose high blood pressure may best be treated surgically, you are now familiar with the sophisticated sequence of diagnostic tests which are required before any decision can be reached about an operation.

The key to the successful control of your high blood pressure is you. It is your body, and only you can ensure that it receives the very best of care. There is no question that the single most important way to improve the overall quality of health care is to "improve the quality of the patient"—and that means you. You and your family are more likely to consistently receive the best care that modern medicine has to offer if you make the effort to inform yourself about health issues and insist that your doctor allow you to share fully in the important decisions that affect your health and the health of those you love.

It is up to you to insist that the initial evaluation of your blood pressure condition be properly performed. The medical interview portion should be extensive. A thorough physical examination can be performed in just a few minutes, but a thorough medical interview takes time. If your doctor seems unwilling or too busy to devote sufficient time to review with you all the important areas outlined in Chapter 5, express your concern. If, instead of reacting positively to your expression of concern, your doctor reacts with anger or assumes an authoritarian attitude, you should consider seeking medical care elsewhere. A defensive attitude is often a sign of insecurity, and it may indicate that your doctor's knowledge about all the issues of high blood pressure is incomplete. At the very least, it suggests a less than complete commitment to helping you take good care of yourself.

Question the unusual. The treatment of high blood pressure has become reasonably standardized, and all physicians should proceed in approximately the same fashion. You should be advised about salt restriction, weight loss, and the benefits of regular physical exercise. Although opinions still differ about the degree of salt restriction that is optimal, *no one should advise you to continue to freely salt your food*. Every effort should be made either to eliminate or reduce all the other risk factors which contribute to diseases of the heart and the blood vessels. *If you smoke, your doctor should take a firm stand and insist that you stop*. Of course, your doctor cannot force you to stop smoking, but even a permissive attitude is unwarranted, because you may interpret it as unspoken approval for you to continue in this destructive habit. If medicines are recommended, they should be introduced in a logical and "stepwise" fashion. Mild medicines should be introduced before strong ones, and the first medicine prescribed should almost always be either a diuretic or one of the beta-blockers. It is estimated that over 50 percent of all individuals who have high blood pressure can be successfully treated with a single medicine taken not more than once or twice a day. Early aggressive treatment with highly potent medication or complex programs is unwarranted (and probably unnecessary) unless your blood pressure elevation is dangerously high. You have every right to expect that treatment will be safe and that side effects will be kept to a minimum, and you should not settle for less.

Your doctor has the tools to safely and effectively bring your blood pressure down to normal, *but only you can keep it there*. Excessive salt intake can counter the effectiveness of medicines. Excessive weight can escalate the quantity of medicine required. The key to the successful control of your high blood pressure is your ongoing commitment to therapy. It is up to you. If salt restriction, weight loss, and regular participation in an exercise program do not completely bring your blood pressure into normal range, it becomes imperative that you take medication on a regular schedule. Extensive, carefully performed studies now clearly demonstrate that adequate control of high blood pressure, no matter how small the initial elevation, dramatically improves both health and longevity. Even a ten-point elevation of pressure above normal should not be allowed. Bringing this very mild elevation of blood pressure back to normal reduces the number of deaths due to heart attack and stroke by nearly 50 percent!

In this age of natural foods and natural methods of health care, many individuals feel that they have somehow failed if they are unable to keep their blood pressure normal without the additional help of a blood pressure medication. More and more individuals are rising up to protest chemical additives, environmental pollutants, and self-destructive attitudes and habits. This is a wholesome movement, and it is hoped that this book will contribute to its growth. However, you should not feel that you have failed because you do find it necessary to take a chemical to bring your blood pressure back to normal and keep it there. Although it is true that science and technology have created problems as well as solutions, it is also true that tools have been developed which, if properly and responsibly employed, improve the quality of life. Medication to treat high blood pressure is one such tool. Certainly you should take advantage of all natural means to prevent blood pressure from rising and to lower it should it go up, but you should not forego the tremendous health benefits which can be yours should medication also be required. This does not indicate a personal failure. It is just another sensible and responsible thing that you and only you can do to take the very best care of your body.

APPENDIX I: Medicines Which May Interact with High Blood Pressure Medication

The following lists will allow you to identify some of the common medicines which can interact importantly with blood pressure medication. In reviewing Chapter 6 for information about your own therapy program you will be able to tell whether any of the names on this list are important to you.

THE TRICYCLIC ANTIDEPRESSANTS

Trade Name • (generic name)

Acelexa • (nortriptyline)
Adepin • (doxepin)
Adepril • (amitriptyline)
Allegron • (nortriptyline)
Altilen • (nortriptyline)
Annolyten • (amitriptyline)
Aponal • (doxepin)
Ateben • (nortriptyline)
Aventyl • (nortriptyline)

Berkomine • (imipramine)

Censtin • (imipramine)
Chemipramine • (imipramine)
Chrytemin • (imipramine)
Curatin • (doxepin)

Demipressin • (imipramine)
Deprex • (amitriptyline)
Deprinol • (imipramine)
Ditisan • (imipraminoxide)
Domical • (amitriptyline)
Doxal • (doxepin)

Doxedyn • (doxepin)
Dynaprin • (imipramine)

Elatrol • (amitriptyline)
Elavil • (amitriptyline)
Elepsin • (imipraminoxide)
Endep • (amitriptyline)
Etraphon • (amitriptyline)

Feinalmin • (imipramine)

IA-Pran • (imipramine)
Imavate • (imipramine)
Imilanyle • (imipramine)
Imiprin • (imipramine)
Imipranil • (imipramine)
Imiprex • (imipraminoxide)
Impranil • (imipramine)
Impril • (imipramine)
Improgen • (imipramine)
Intalpram • (imipramine)
Iramil • (imipramine)

Janimine • (imipramine)

THE TRICYCLIC ANTIDEPRESSANTS *(continued)*

Laroxal • (amitriptyline)
Laroxyl • (amitriptyline)
Larozyl • (amitriptyline)
Lentizol • (amitriptyline)
Levate • (amitriptyline)
Limbitrol • (amitriptyline)

Mareline • (amitriptyline)
Maximed • (protriptyline)
Melipramin • (imipramine)
Meripramin • (imipramine)

Nebril • (desipramine)
Norpolake • (desipramine)
Norpramine • (desipramine)
Nortab • (nortriptyline)
Nortimil • (desipramine)
Nortrilen • (nortriptyline)
Norzepine • (nortriptyline)
Novopramine • (imipramine)
Novotriptyn • (amitriptyline)
Novoxapin • (doxepin)

Pamelor • (nortriptyline)
Pertofran • (desipramine)
Pertofrane • (desipramine)
Pertofrina • (desipramine)
Presamine • (imipramine)
Pryleugan • (imipramine)

Psychoforin • (imipramine)
Psychostyl • (nortriptyline)

Redomex • (amitriptyline)

Saroten • (amitriptyline)
Sarotex • (amitriptyline)
Sensaval • (nortriptyline)
Sensival • (nortriptyline)
Sertofren • (desipramine)
Sinequan • (doxepin)
Sinquan • (doxepin)
SK-Pramine • (imipramine)
Surmontil • (trimipramine)
Surplix • (imipramine)

Teperin • (imipramine)
Tofranil • (imipramine)
Tofranil-PM • (imipramine)
Toruan • (doxepin)
Triavil • (amitriptyline)
Triptil • (protriptyline)
Triptyl • (amitriptyline)
Tryptacap • (amitriptyline)
Tryptanol • (amitriptyline)
Tryptizol • (amitriptyline)

Vivactil • (protriptyline)
Vividyl • (nortriptyline)

THE PHENOTHIAZINES

Trade Name • (generic name)

Adazine • (triflupromazine)
Anatensol • (fluphenazine)
Anti-naus • (prochlorperazine)
Aphilan • (buclizine)
Atarzine • (promazine)

Brotopon • (haloperidol)
Buclifen • (buclizine)
Buclina • (buclizine)

Calmansial • (fluphenazine)
Calmazine • (trifluoperazine)
Centractyl • (promazine)
Chemflurazine • (trifluoperazine)
Chloractil • (chlorpromazine)
Chlorazin • (chlorpromazine)

Chlorpernazine • (prochlorperazine)
Chlorpromados • (chlorpromazine)
Chlor-Promanyl • (chlorpromazine)
Chlorprom-Ez-Etz • (chlorpromazine)
Chlor-PZ • (chlorpromazine)
Clinazine • (trifluoperazine)
Compazine • (prochlorperazine)
Cromedazine • (chlorpromazine)

Dapotum • (fluphenazine)
Dapotum D • (fluphenazine)
Daxolin • (loxapine)
Decentin • (perphenazine)

Elmarine • (chlorpromazine)
Eskazinyl • (trifluoperazine)
Esmind • (chlorpromazine)
Eutimux • (fluphenazine)

THE PHENOTHIAZINES *(continued)*

Fenactil • (chlorpromazine)
Fentazin • (perphenazine)
Fluazine • (trifluoperazine)
Fluomazina • (triflupromazine)
Fluropen • (triflupromazine)
F-Mon • (perphenazine)
Frenil • (promazine)

Haldol • (haloperidol)
Hibernal • (chlorpromazine)
Hibernil • (chlorpromazine)
Histabutazine • (buclizine)

Intrazine • (promazine)

Jatroneurol • (trifluoperazine)

Keselan • (haloperidol)
Klometil • (prochloroperazine)
Klorazine • (chlorpromazine)
Klorproman • (chlorpromazine)
Klorpromex • (chlorpromazine)

Largactil • (chlorpromazine)
Lidanar • (mesoridazine)
Lidanil • (mesoridazine)
Lidanol • (mesoridazine)
Longifene • (buclizine)
Loxapal • (loxapine)
Loxitane • (loxapine)
Lyogen • (fluphenazine)
Lyorodin • (fluphenazine)

Mallorol • (thioridazine)
Mefid • (perphenazine)
Megalectil • (butaperazine)
Megaphen • (chlorpromazine)
Mellaril • (thioridazine)
Melleretten • (thioridazine)
Melleril • (thioridazine)
Minithixen • (chlorprothine)
Mirenil • (fluphenazine)
Moditen • (fluphenazine)
Mopan • (molindane)

Navane • (thiothixene)
Neurazine • (chlorpromazine)
Neuriplege • (chlorprethazine)
Neuronal • (butaperazine)
Nipodal • (prochlorperazine)
Nivoman • (triflupromazine)
Novoflurazine • (trifluoperazine)
Novoridazine • (thioridazine)

Omca • (fluphenazine)
Ornazine • (chlorpromazine)
Orsanil • (thioridazine)

Pacinol • (fluphenazine)
Pentazine • (trifluoperazine)
Peratsin • (perphenazine)
Permitil • (fluphenazine)
Postafen • (buclizine)
Prazine • (promazine)
Proketazine • (carphenazine)
Prolixin • (fluphenazine)
Promachel • (chlorpromazine)
Promachlor • (chlorpromazine)
Promacid • (chlorpromazine)
Promanyl • (promazine)
Promapar • (chlorpromazine)
Promazettes • (promazine)
Promexin • (chlorpromazine)
Promezerine • (promazine)
Promosol • (chlorpromazine)
Prophaphenin • (chlorpromazine)
Protactyl • (promazine)
Pro-Tran • (promazine)
Prozil • (chlorpromazine)
Psylaktil • (chlorpromazine)
Psymod • (piperacetazine)
Psyquil • (triflupromazine)

Quide • (piperacetazine)

Repoise • (butaperazine)
Retamine • (buclizine)

Sediston • (promazine)
Serenace • (haloperidol)
Serentil • (mesoridazine)
Sevinol • (fluphenazine)
Siqualone • (fluphenazine)
Siquil • (triflupromazine)
Softran • (buclizine)
Solazine • (trifluoperazine)
Sonazine • (chlorpromazine)
Sparine • (promazine)
Starazine • (promazine)
Stelazine • (trifluoperazine)
Stemetil • (prochlorperazine)

Talofen • (promazine)
Taractan • (chlorprothixene)
Tarasan • (chlorprothixene)
Tementil • (prochlorperazine)
Terfluzine • (trifluoperazine)
Thioril • (thioridazine)

THE PHENOTHIAZINES *(continued)*

Thorazine • (chlorpromazine)
Tindal • (acetophenazine)
Tindala • (acetophenazine)
Trancin • (fluphenazine)
Trifluoper-Ez-Etz • (trifluoperazine)
Triflurin • (trifluoperazine)
Trilafan • (perphenazine)
Trilafon • (perphenazine)
Truxal • (chlorprothixene)

Truxaletter • (chlorprothixene)
Tyrylen • (butaperazine)

Verophen • (promazine)
Vertigon • (prochlorperazine)
Vesporal • (triflupromazine)
Vesprin • (triflupromazine)
Vibazine • (buclizine)

THE MONOAMINE OXIDASE INHIBITORS

Trade Name • (generic name)

Eatonyl • (pargyline)

Furoxone • (furazolidone)

Ludiomil • (mebanazine)

Marplan • (isocarboxazide)

Marsalid • (iproniazide)

Nardelzine • (phenelzine)
Nardil • (phenelzine)
Niamide • (nialamide)

Parnate • (tranylcypromine)

THE LITHIUM COMPOUNDS

Lithium acetate:
- Quilonorm
- Quilonum

Lithium carbonate:

Carbolith	Lithionate	Lito
Eskalith	Lithium Oligosol	Manialith
Eutimin	Lithizine	Maniprex
Hypnorex	Litho-Carb	Neurolepsin
Licarb	Lithotabs	Pfi-Lithium
Lithane	Liticar	Phasal
Lithea	Litin	Plenur
Lithicarb		Priadel

Lithium citrate:
- Demalit
- Litarex

Lithium sulfate:
Lithiofor
Lithionit
Lithium-Duriles

APPENDIX II:
Advice To Travelers

If you are taking medication to control high blood pressure, you should be aware that not all medicines are available in every country and that it is usually very difficult for a physician or pharmacist (chemist) in one country to identify the nature of a medicine prescribed by a physician elsewhere. Accordingly, if you intend to travel abroad, you should plan to pack enough medicine to last the entire trip. On the chance that any of your medication should be lost or its supply become exhausted during your travels, the information presented here will show you how to obtain a replacement safely.

You will remember that most medicines are known by two names, trade and generic (chemical). A medicine may have many trade names, but it has only one generic name. The generic name of a medicine is an international designation of its chemical structure. This designation is the same in all countries. The trade name of a medicine is a brand name, designed for quick identification, easy recall, and maximizing sales. Unlike generic names, the trade name of a medicine may differ in different countries, even those nations sharing a common language. There are two major reasons for this. First, a medicine which is sold by one pharmaceutical firm in one country may be sold by a different elsewhere. Should this be the case, the trade name of the medicine will vary by country since companies have exclusive rights to the trade names they choose for a medicine. Secondly, even if a medicine is manufactured by the *same* firm, its trade name is likely to change from country to country, because a name which sounds appealing in one language may have little attraction in another.

Doctors usually prescribe medicines by their trade names which are easier to remember and write. Yet it is the generic name you will probably need to know should you find it necessary to obtain a replacement for one of your medicines while abroad. Doctors and pharmacists (chemists) are usually able to identify a foreign medication when given the generic name but are generally unable to do so by trade name alone. Available reference materials only provide information about medicines which are sold in a given country. The expense of incorporating trade names used abroad into local source materials seldom justifies the limited usage to which such listings would be put. The International Medicine Index is designed to overcome this problem.

By using this Index, it should be possible for a physician or pharmacist (chemist) abroad to dispense to you exactly the same medicine which you are taking at home. It is quite likely that its trade name will vary by country but as long as the generic name is the same, the medicine will be identical. Of course you must know the dosage so that you can be sure that you receive not only the correct medication but also the proper amount. Suppose for example you are an American, take 0.2 mg of Naqua daily to control your blood pressure, and are visiting in France. While there, you run out of your medicine. By looking in the International Medicine Index, you learn that Naqua is the trade name for trichlormethiazide (page 80). With this information, a physician or pharmacist (chemist) can give you 0.2 mg of Fluitran, which is the trade name used in France for trichlormethiazide. If you wish to double check to make sure that you have been given the correct medicine, you can look up Fluitran in the International Medicine Index to confirm that its generic name is trichlormethiazide (page 79). Thus the Index not only provides the generic name of all your blood pressure medicine; it also confirms the reliability and accuracy of the people from whom you seek help.

Remember that fixed combination medicines have two or more generic names, one for each of the medicines in the combination. For example, if you look up Combipres 0.1, in the International Medicine Index, you will learn that it is a combination of chlorthalidone 15 mg and clonidine 0.1 mg (page 87). It may turn out that Combipres 0.1 is unavailable as an equivalent fixed combination medicine in the country which you are visiting because like trade names, fixed combination medicines tend not to travel. However, both chlorthalidone and clonidine are available as separate medicines in almost every part of the world. Thus, if you require a replacement for Combipres 0.1, you should be able to make an exact substitution by requesting chlorthalidone 0.15 mg plus clonidine 0.1 mg. Your blood pressure will be as well controlled by taking each component separately as by taking them in fixed combination. It is quite likely that each of the substitute medicines you are given in the above case will have a trade name. By looking these trade names up in the International Medicine Index you will be able to confirm that the medicines you have received are in fact chlorthalidone and clonidine.

What if the medicine you are taking is simply not available

in the country you are visiting? This is sometimes the case with the newer high blood pressure medicines. It is expensive for a pharmaceutical firm to introduce a new medicine into a country, and often the firm will concentrate its marketing efforts on one country at the start. This can create real problems, because even if you know the generic name of your medicine, a foreign physician or pharmacist (chemist) may be unable to identify it in order to make a rational substitution. Their reference material will not list either the generic *or* the trade name of medicines which are not sold in that country. This problem, too, is overcome by the International Medicine Index as we shall see shortly.

All the medicines which are used to treat high blood pressure can be arranged into groups, such as diuretics and beta-blockers. All the medicines within a particular group are essentially equivalent. Consequently, if your medicine is unavailable in the country in which you are visiting, a local physician or pharmacist (chemist) should be able to recommend a safe and equally effective substitute once it is known to which *group* your medicine belongs. The information in this book is so arranged that it becomes easy to identify the group to which a medicine belongs so that another with similar properties can be substituted. Either the trade name or the generic name can be used for this purpose. An example will make this clear.

Suppose you live in the United Kingdom, take 80 mg of Trasicor once daily, and travel to the United States. While there, you run out of your medicine. The Index shows that Trasicor is the trade name of oxprenolol. The Index reference also indicates that oxprenolol belongs to the group of beta-blockers. When you request more oxprenolol from an American physician (in the United States blood pressure medicines can only be obtained upon written prescription of a physician), you will be informed that this medicine is unavailable in the United States. However, because you are also able to inform the physician that your medicine is one of the beta-blockers, the physician can at least supply you with a medicine from the same group. In fact, if you take this back with you, the physician will be able to look over the section on beta-blockers in order to decide which one of the beta-blockers available in America has properties most like your oxprenolol (page 75). Three beta-blockers are currently available in America: propranolol, metoprolol, and nadolol. The information in this book will allow the physician to learn that both metoprolol (page 75) and nadolol (page 75) more closely resemble oxprenolol than does propranolol (page 72). Consequently, the best choice is to give you either 50 mg or 100 mg of metoprolol to take twice daily or 160 mg of nadolol to take once daily. Either choice will safely and effectively substitute for your medicine until you return home.

It could happen that a foreign physician would recommend medication quite different from that which you have been using. This could be excellent medical advice. You may well want to try such a new treatment program and the International Medicine Index can help locate and inform you about any new medication to be sure that the advice you've been given is medically sound and that there are no undesirable side effects, important drug interactions, or warnings involved.

Finally, the International Medicine Index allows you to protect yourself in the event that a physician or pharmacist (chemist) abroad gives you inappropriate medication. By consulting the Index you can identify a high blood pressure medicine once you know either its trade or generic name. Either the medicine should be chemically identical to your former medicine (same generic name) or it should be a rational substitution (similar mechanism of action and similar side effects). It is extremely important that the medicine which is substituted does not interact adversely with other medicine you may be taking and that it not have the potential of adversely affecting any medical condition you may have. The information in Chapter Seven makes it possible for you to guard against either of these possibilities. And remember: *Do not accept any medicine that you cannot identify. If the medicine is dispensed in an unmarked container, do not accept it. Ask that the name be added. If the person supplying your medicine is unable or unwilling to do this, refuse the medicine.*

International Medicine Index

While there are actually a relatively small number of medicines that are employed in the treatment of high blood pressure, there are a multitude of trade names, because many different pharmaceutical firms manufacture the same medicine, each under a different trade name. The International Medicine Index will allow you quickly to identify high blood pressure medication wherever you may be. It also gives the page numbers for the "potassium-sparing agents" and potassium supplements which are described in Chapter 8.

Medicines that are used throughout the world are included on this list, although not all the medicines are available in every country. For example, many medicines are not available in the United States either because the manufacturers have not requested approval of the Federal Drug Administration or because such approval is still pending. The fact that a medicine is not available in one country but is available in another should not be taken to indicate that there might be something wrong with the medicine. Complex licensing regulations as well as marketing decisions of the pharmaceutical firms influence what medicine will be sold where.

General Index